# Intermittent Fasting

# Secret to Fabulous 50 and Over:

## The Metabolic Reset, Weight Loss, Energy Boost, Memory Improvement, and Healthy Lifestyle Benefits of Intermittent Fasting for Women Over 50

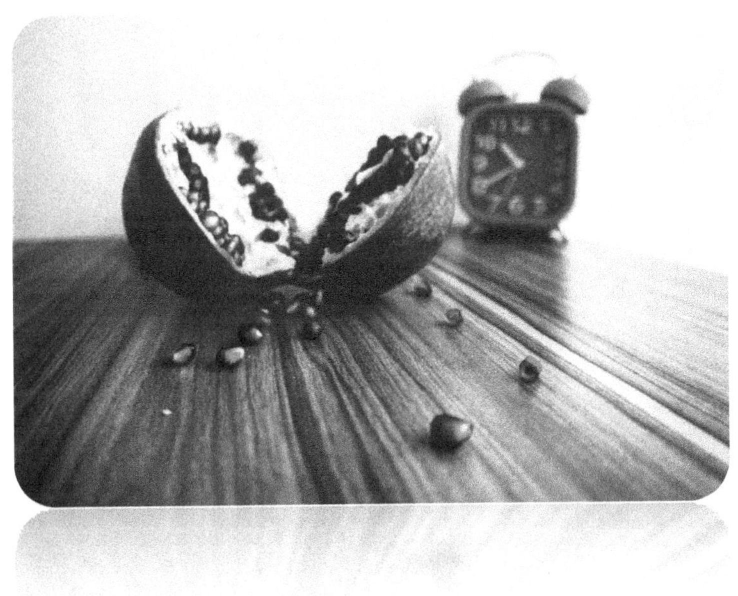

**Teresa J. Allen**

# Table of Contents

# Introduction

## Understanding Intermittent Fasting

Intermittent fasting, a dietary strategy that alternates times of eating with periods of fasting, has attracted increasing interest in recent years for its potential health advantages. In this book, "Intermittent Fasting for Women Over 50: Reset Your Metabolism, Lose Weight, Boost Your Energy, Improve Memory, and Enjoy a Healthy Life," we go into the intricacies of intermittent fasting specifically targeted for women over the Age of 50.

Understanding the physiological changes that occur as women age is crucial to designing successful health solutions. As women reach menopause and beyond, hormonal oscillations, changes in metabolism, and modifications in body composition become increasingly prominent. These changes might pose distinct problems to maintaining a healthy weight, controlling energy levels, and sustaining cognitive function.

## Why Intermittent Fasting Works for Women Over 50

Intermittent fasting offers a promising way to address these difficulties. By properly scheduling periods of eating and fasting, individuals can tap into the body's natural systems for energy control, metabolic flexibility, and cellular repair. For women over 50, intermittent fasting holds particular appeal due to its potential to reset metabolic function, assist weight loss, boost energy levels, enhance cognitive function, and promote general well-being.

The science underlying intermittent fasting is founded in the body's response to periods of food deprivation, a state that generates a cascade of metabolic modifications geared at survival. During fasting times, insulin levels decline, prompting the body to utilize stored fat for energy. This metabolic shift not only improves fat reduction but also enhances insulin sensitivity, a vital role in preventing type 2 diabetes and metabolic syndrome, illnesses that become increasingly prevalent with age.

## Benefits of Intermittent Fasting for Women Over 50

Moreover, intermittent fasting has been proven to induce autophagy, a cellular mechanism that eliminates damaged components and promotes cellular rejuvenation. This procedure is particularly essential for women over 50, since it may help offset age-related decreases in cellular function and minimize the risk of chronic diseases such as Alzheimer's, Parkinson's, and cardiovascular disease.

In this book, we will study the scientific concepts underlying intermittent fasting and its specific applications for women over 50. We will go into the many ways of intermittent fasting, examine tactics for meal planning and nutrition, address frequent obstacles and traps, and provide practical ideas for incorporating intermittent fasting into daily life. Additionally, we will discuss the role of exercise, tracking progress, and the long-term health implications of intermittent fasting.

It is crucial to remember that while intermittent fasting offers various potential benefits, it may not be ideal for everyone, especially those with certain medical issues or individual dietary demands. As such, we advise speaking with a healthcare expert before embarking on any fasting regimen, particularly for women over 50 who may have unique health considerations.

In summary, this book provides as a thorough guide to leveraging the potential of intermittent fasting to maximize health, vitality, and longevity for women over 50. By learning the science underlying intermittent fasting and following evidence-based practices, readers may embark on a journey towards resetting their metabolism, achieving sustained weight loss, raising energy levels, enhancing memory, and enjoying a healthier, more satisfying life.

# Chapter 1

# Intermittent Fasting: A Scientific Overview

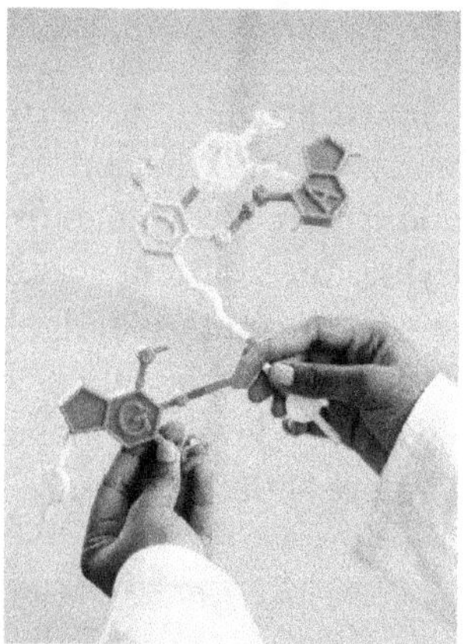

## How Intermittent Fasting Affects Your Metabolism

Metabolism, the sum of all biochemical processes within the body, is a complex interplay of energy production, consumption, and storage. Intermittent fasting, characterized by alternating periods of eating and fasting, exerts dramatic effects on metabolism through numerous mechanisms that involve energy substrates, hormones, and cellular signaling pathways.

**Energy Substrate Utilization:** Intermittent fasting promotes considerable alterations in energy substrate usage, particularly during fasting periods. Without dietary glucose, the body draws into stored energy stores to meet metabolic demands. Initially, glycogen stores, largely held in the liver and muscles, are mobilized to sustain blood glucose levels. However, as fasting continues, glycogen stores become depleted, leading to a switch to fat metabolism.

This metabolic switch from glucose to fat metabolism is assisted by decreased insulin levels and increased glucagon release, a hormone that stimulates fat breakdown (lipolysis) and ketogenesis, the generation of ketone molecules from fatty acids. Ketone bodies, such as beta-hydroxybutyrate and acetoacetate, serve as alternate fuel sources for tissues, including the brain, muscles, and heart, during fasting periods. This condition of elevated ketone generation, known as ketosis, is a hallmark of intermittent fasting and is associated with greater metabolic flexibility and energy efficiency.

**Hormonal Regulation:** Intermittent fasting produces dramatic impacts on hormone secretion and signaling networks that regulate metabolism, hunger, and energy balance. One of the primary hormonal changes generated by fasting is a drop in insulin levels. Insulin, released by the pancreas in response to dietary carbs, stimulates glucose uptake and storage in tissues and inhibits fat breakdown. During fasting times, insulin levels drop, leading to enhanced lipolysis, fat oxidation, and ketogenesis.

Conversely, intermittent fasting enhances the release of growth hormone (GH), a peptide hormone that plays a critical role in metabolism, growth, and tissue repair. GH increases fat mobilization, muscular development, and protein synthesis, hence conserving lean body mass during fasting times. Moreover, GH promotes insulin sensitivity and glucose uptake in peripheral tissues, further contributing to metabolic health and energy use.

Additionally, intermittent fasting alters the release of other hormones involved in hunger regulation, such as ghrelin and leptin. Ghrelin, produced by the stomach, is known as the "hunger hormone" because it stimulates appetite and promotes food intake. Fasting increases ghrelin secretion, resulting in temporary feelings of hunger that normally fade over time. In contrast, leptin, produced by adipose tissue, functions as a satiety signal that decreases appetite and regulates energy expenditure. Intermittent fasting may promote leptin sensitivity, leading to enhanced appetite control and reduced calorie consumption.

**Cellular Signaling Pathways:** Intermittent fasting activates multiple cellular signaling pathways that govern metabolism, cellular repair, and stress resistance. One of the primary mechanisms implicated in the metabolic impacts of fasting is the adenosine monophosphate-activated protein kinase (AMPK) pathway. AMPK is a cellular energy sensor that becomes activated in response to low-energy situations, such as fasting or exercise. Activated AMPK enhances energy production by boosting glucose uptake, fatty acid oxidation, and mitochondrial biogenesis while suppressing energy-consuming processes such as protein synthesis and cell growth.

Furthermore, intermittent fasting stimulates autophagy, a cellular recycling process that eliminates damaged or defective cellular components and promotes cellular renewal and repair. Autophagy is enhanced during fasting periods as a technique of conserving energy and optimizing cellular function. By sweeping out accumulated junk and damaged organelles, autophagy helps maintain cellular homeostasis and reduce age-related losses in metabolic activity.

In summary, intermittent fasting produces dramatic impacts on metabolism through numerous processes involving energy substrate use, hormone control, and cellular signaling pathways. By boosting fat metabolism, enhancing insulin sensitivity, and triggering cellular repair mechanisms, intermittent fasting delivers metabolic benefits that may contribute to enhanced metabolic health, weight control, and lifespan.

## Hormonal Changes and Their Impact on Weight Loss: The Roller Coaster Ride Inside Your Body

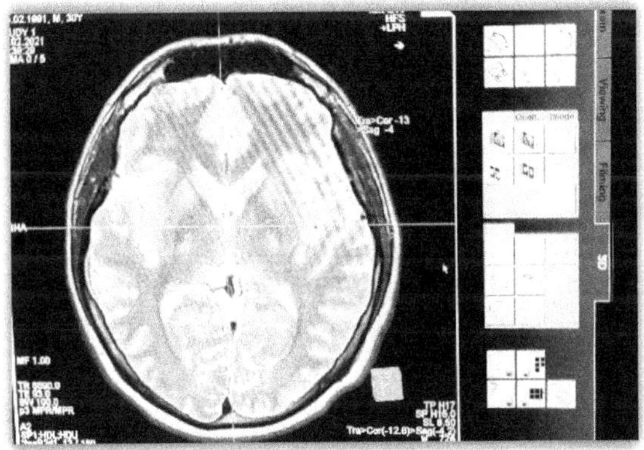

Buckle up, because we're about to take a wild voyage through the hormonal terrain of weight loss! Hormones are like the conductors of a symphony orchestra inside your body, organizing everything from hunger cues to energy consumption. When it comes to removing those obstinate pounds, understanding how these hormonal maestros wield their batons can make all the difference in your weight loss journey.

**Insulin:** The Glucose Gatekeeper First up, we have insulin, the gatekeeper of glucose. Produced by your pancreas, insulin's principal purpose is to transfer glucose from your bloodstream into your cells for energy or storage. However, when you're continuously noshing on sugary snacks and carb-laden treats, insulin goes into overdrive, leading to insulin resistance and fat storage.

Enter intermittent fasting, the hero of our narrative! By giving your body, a break from regular eating, intermittent fasting helps lower insulin levels, allowing your cells to become more sensitive to its effects. This means less fat storage and greater fat burning, leading to a smaller waistline and happy hormones.

**Ghrelin and Leptin:** The Hunger Heroes Next, we have ghrelin and leptin, the dynamic duet of hunger regulation. Ghrelin, fondly known as the "hunger hormone," is like your body's natural alarm clock, alerting you when it's time to recharge. Meanwhile, leptin, the "satiety hormone," touches you on the shoulder and whispers, "Hey, you've had enough."

But what happens when these hormones become out of sync? Cue the late-night food attacks and bottomless pit syndrome! Intermittent fasting comes to the rescue once again, helping reset your hunger hormones and restore harmony to your appetite. With fewer hunger pangs and improved portion control, you'll find sticking to your weight loss objectives easier than ever.

**Cortisol:** The Stress Monster Last but not least, we have cortisol, the stress monster lurking in the shadows. When stress levels climb, cortisol levels follow suit, triggering a cascade of hormonal turmoil that can wreak havoc on your waistline. Not only does cortisol increase fat storage, particularly around the abdomen, but it also drives up your desire for all things sweet and salty.

Luckily, intermittent fasting has a special weapon against cortisol: resilience! By practicing mindfulness, getting plenty of sleep, and including stress-reducing activities like yoga or meditation into your routine, you may keep cortisol in check and avoid it from derailing your weight loss attempts.

So there you have it, guys! Hormonal shifts may feel like a chaotic roller coaster ride at times, but with intermittent fasting as your trusted guide, you can negotiate the twists and turns with ease. By leveraging the power of insulin management, hunger hormone harmony, and stress resilience, you'll unlock the key to sustainable weight loss and a happier, healthier self. So climb onboard the intermittent fasting express and get ready to enjoy the experience of a lifetime!

# Metabolic Benefits for Women Over 50: Unlocking Your Full Potential

Welcome to the age of empowerment, when women over 50 are rewriting the norms and regaining their energy like never before! In this chapter, we'll explore the metabolic miracles of intermittent fasting and how it may improve your life from the inside out.

**Resetting Your Metabolic Clock:** As we journey through life, our metabolic rate tends to slow down, like a worn engine striving to keep up with the demands of daily existence. But who says we have to accept this as our fate? Intermittent fasting offers a refreshing reset button for your metabolic clock, giving your body a much-needed break from incessant eating and allowing it to readjust and regenerate.

By including intervals of fasting into your regimen, you're essentially giving your metabolism a chance to catch its breath and enhance its effectiveness. This can lead to a range of benefits, including higher fat burning, improved insulin sensitivity, and enhanced metabolic flexibility. So say goodbye to sluggish metabolisms and welcome to a revived, energized you!

**Shedding Those Stubborn Pounds:** Let's face it, weight reduction may be a problem at any age, but it can feel especially daunting as we hit our fifth decade and beyond. However, intermittent fasting gives a glimpse of hope in the battle against obstinate pounds. By increasing fat loss while keeping lean muscle mass, intermittent fasting helps you accomplish lasting weight loss without compromising your hard-earned                              muscle                              tone.

Moreover, intermittent fasting has been demonstrated to target visceral fat, the harmful fat that collects around your organs and raises your risk of chronic diseases including heart disease and type 2 diabetes. So not only will you look and feel better, but you'll also be defending your long-term health in the                                                                    process.

**Boosting Energy Levels:** Who says energy levels have to drop as we age? With intermittent fasting as your secret weapon, you'll be humming with vitality and enthusiasm from sunrise to sunset! By optimizing energy production and use, intermittent fasting helps erase those mid-afternoon slumps and keeps you feeling sharp, focused, and awake throughout the day.

Plus, intermittent fasting has been demonstrated to boost mitochondrial function, the powerhouses of your cells responsible for creating energy. By promoting mitochondrial health and efficiency, intermittent fasting guarantees that your body has a continuous source of energy to fuel your daily activities, from morning workouts to afternoon meetings to evening social engagements.

**Improving Cognitive Function:** Memory lapses and brain fog get you feeling like you're caught in a mental rut. Not to worry, since intermittent fasting is here to offer your brain a much-needed boost! Studies have indicated that intermittent fasting can promote cognitive performance, improve memory, and protect against age-related neurodegenerative disorders like Alzheimer's.

But how does intermittent fasting work its magic on the brain? One notion is that fasting triggers the creation of brain-derived neurotrophic factor (BDNF), a protein that supports the growth and repair of neurons. By boosting the creation of BDNF, intermittent fasting helps keep your brain bright, agile, and robust, helping you to stay mentally sharp far into your golden years.

**Embracing a Healthier, Happier You:** At the end of the day, it's not just about the numbers on the scale or the inches around your waist. It's about restoring your health, vigor, and zest for life. With intermittent fasting as your trusted companion, you'll not only look better, but you'll also feel great from the inside out, radiating confidence, joy, and energy wherever you go.

So go on, embrace your inner powerhouse, and release the entire potential that's been waiting inside you all along. With intermittent fasting as your guidance, the sky's the limit, and the best is yet to come!

# Chapter 2

# Getting Started with Intermittent Fasting

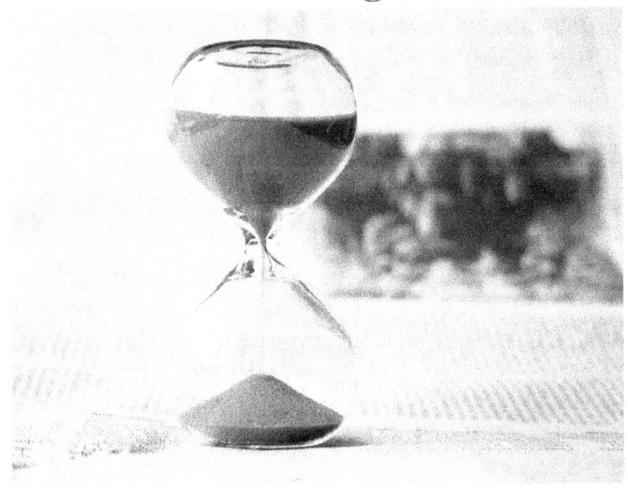

## Choosing the Right Intermittent Fasting Plan: Your Personalized Path to Success

Hey there, intrepid adventurers on the quest to better health and wellness! As you walk into the domain of intermittent fasting, you may find yourself faced with an enticing assortment of fasting programs, each promising to uncover the key to your ultimate well-being. But worry not, because we're here to be your reliable guides as you explore this thrilling territory and discover the intermittent fasting strategy that's suited for you!

**The 16/8 Method: The Goldilocks of Fasting** Plans

First up, we have the 16/8 method, sometimes known as the "time-restricted eating" approach. This fasting schedule is like the Goldilocks of intermittent fasting - not too rigorous, not too lenient, but just suitable for many novices and seasoned fasters alike. With the 16/8 technique, you'll fast for 16 hours each day and restrict you're eating window to 8 hours, leaving plenty of time for your body to gain the metabolic benefits of fasting without feeling deprived or hungry.

But don't let the simplicity of the 16/8 technique deceive you - it delivers a tremendous punch when it comes to weight loss, metabolic health, and overall well-being. By giving your body a break from constant eating and letting it tap into stored fat for energy, the 16/8 technique can help you shed stubborn pounds, raise energy levels, and improve insulin sensitivity, all while enjoying great, fulfilling meals during your eating window.

**The 5:2 Method: Feast and Famine, with a Twist**

Next on our list is the 5:2 technique, a fasting strategy that adds a splash of excitement to your weekly routine. With the 5:2 technique, you'll eat normally for five days of the week and then limit your calorie intake to 500-600 calories on two non-consecutive days. It's like a tiny journey in feast and famine, with a twist!

While the 5:2 method may appear a bit more demanding than the 16/8 approach, many individuals find it to be a flexible and sustainable way to include intermittent fasting into their routine. Plus, the rare fast days can provide a nice change from the monotony of everyday meals and allow your body a chance to reset and renew.

## Alternate Day Fasting: A Roller Coaster Ride for Your Metabolism

If you're searching for a fasting schedule that's a bit more daring, go no further than alternate-day fasting! With this strategy, you'll alternate between fasting days, where you consume extremely few calories or none at all, and feast days, where you eat to your heart's content. It's like a roller coaster trip for your metabolism, with plenty of twists and turns along the way!

While alternate-day fasting may not be for the faint of heart, it can give impressive benefits when it comes to weight loss, metabolic health, and longevity. By challenging your body with times of fasting and feasting, alternate-day fasting can help increase insulin sensitivity, stimulate fat burning, and promote cellular repair and regeneration.

## Extended Fasting: The Ultimate Test of Endurance

Last but not least, we have prolonged fasting, the ultimate test of endurance for seasoned fasters eager to push their boundaries and uncover the full potential of intermittent fasting. With extended fasting, you'll fast for periods ranging from 24 hours to several days or even weeks, allowing your body to enter a state of severe ketosis and experience substantial metabolic and cellular changes.

While lengthy fasting may sound scary, many people find it to be a transformative experience that leads to remarkable gains in weight loss, metabolic health, and overall well-being. Plus, the mental clarity, spiritual insights, and sense of success that come with finishing an extended fast can be truly empowering and life-changing.

So, there you have it, fellow travelers! Whether you're drawn to the simplicity of the 16/8 method, the excitement of the 5:2 approach, the adventure of alternate-day fasting, or the challenge of extended fasting, there's an intermittent fasting strategy out there that's right for you. So go ahead, research your alternatives, and go on the journey to greater health and wellness with confidence and joy!

## Setting Realistic Goals for Women Over 50: Crafting Your Personalized Path to Vitality

Hey there, amazing females over 50 who are eager to go on a path of transformation and regeneration! As you dive into the world of intermittent fasting with the goal of resetting your metabolism, shedding those stubborn pounds, boosting your energy levels, enhancing your memory, and enjoying a vibrant, healthy life, it's time to roll up your sleeves and set some goals that are as bold and beautiful as you are. But fret not, because we're here to be your loyal companions as you negotiate this adventurous terrain and pave the route for your ultimate achievement!

**Define Your Why:** Igniting the Flame of Motivation

Picture this you wake up each morning feeling invigorated, lively, and ready to take on the world. You smoothly glide into your favorite jeans, your memory is sharp as a pin, and you're radiating with confidence and vitality. Sounds like a dream, right? Well, guess what? With intermittent fasting as your faithful friend, your dream can become your reality!

But first, let's get down to the heart of the matter and ask yourself: why do you wish to begin on this journey? Is it to recapture your youthful energy, feel more confident in your skin, or simply have a healthier, more vibrant life? Whatever your reason may be, understanding your "why" is the gasoline that will light the flame of inspiration and carry you forward, especially when the going gets rough.

## Be Specific and Measurable: Painting Your Portrait of Success

Now that you've got your "why" firmly in place, it's time to get down to business and make your goals as explicit and measurable as possible. Instead of saying, "I want to lose weight," try saying, "I want to lose 10 pounds in the next three months." By setting clear, concrete goals that you can track and measure over time, you'll not only stay focused and motivated, but you'll also be able to celebrate your progress and success along the way.

## Break it Down: Taking One Step at a Time

As the saying goes, Rome wasn't built in a day, and neither are your objectives! Instead of trying to handle everything at once, break your goals down into smaller, more doable tasks that you can tackle one at a time. Whether it's starting with a 12-hour fasting window and gradually working your way up to 16 hours, or introducing one new healthy habit into your routine each week, taking modest, consistent steps is the key to long-term success.

## Be Realistic and Flexible: Embracing the Journey

Life is like a box of chocolates - you never know what you're going to get! While it's good to set lofty goals that push you out of your comfort zone, it's also important to be realistic and adaptable in your approach. Understand that failures and problems are a natural part of any journey, and be open to adapting your goals and expectations accordingly. Remember, progress, not perfection, is the name of the game!

**Celebrate Your Wins: You've Earned It!**

Last but not least, don't forget to enjoy your wins along the way! Whether it's reaching a milestone on the scale, adhering to your fasting plan for a week straight, or noticing improvements in your energy levels and memory, take the time to slap yourself on the back and relish in your accomplishments. After all, you've worked hard for it, and you deserve to revel in the glory of your accomplishment!

So, there you have it, gorgeous ladies over 50! Whether you're looking to reset your metabolism, reduce weight, raise your energy levels, improve your memory, or simply enjoy a healthier, more vibrant life with intermittent fasting, setting realistic objectives is the key to making your aspirations become reality. So, think big, start small, and take action now the world is yours for the taking!


## Preparing Mentally and Physically for Intermittent Fasting: Gear Up for Your Wellness Adventure!

Hey there, wellness warriors and adventurous spirits! As you gear up to go on the exhilarating voyage of intermittent fasting, it's time to stretch those mental and physical muscles and prepare yourself for the experience of a lifetime. But fret not, for we're here to be your reliable guides as you navigate this thrilling territory and discover the potential of intermittent fasting to improve your body, mind, and spirit!

## Understand the Basics: Knowledge is Power

First things first, let's get down to the nitty-gritty and learn the foundations of intermittent fasting. In a nutshell, intermittent fasting includes alternating periods of eating and fasting, allowing your body to dip into stored fat for energy and reap a plethora of health benefits, from weight loss and improved metabolic health to enhanced cognitive function and                                                                    longevity.

But worry not, because intermittent fasting is not as scary as it may appear! With a little bit of education and preparation, you'll be well-equipped to embrace this transforming lifestyle with confidence and joy.

## Start Slow and Ease Into It: Rome Wasn't Built in a Day

Now that you've got the basics down, it's time to ease into intermittent fasting and give your body time to acclimate. Rome wasn't built in a day, and neither is your fasting habit! Instead of rushing headfirst into a 16-hour fasting window, start slow and progressively extend the duration of your fasts over time.

Consider starting with a 12-hour fasting window and progressively working your way up to 14, 16, or even 18 hours, depending on your comfort level and individual needs. By taking things gradually and listening to your body's cues, you'll offer yourself the best chance of success and avoid feeling overwhelmed or disheartened.

## Stay Hydrated and Nourished: Fuel Your Body, Fuel Your Adventure

As you embark on your intermittent fasting adventure, it's crucial to stay hydrated and nourished to support your body's needs. While you may be tempted to go for a snack or a sugary drink during fasting periods, opt for water, herbal tea, or black coffee instead to stay hydrated and keep hunger away.

During your eating window, focus on fueling your body with nutrient-dense foods that provide sustained energy and support overall health and well-being. Load up on fruits, veggies, lean proteins, whole grains, and healthy fats to fuel your journey and keep you feeling satisfied and motivated throughout the day.

## Practice Mindfulness and Self-Care: Nurture Your Mind, Body, and Spirit

As you negotiate the ups and downs of intermittent fasting, it's crucial to focus on mindfulness and self-care to nurture your mind, body, and spirit. Take time each day to practice relaxation techniques such as deep breathing, meditation, or gentle stretching to reduce stress and develop a sense of peace and balance.

Additionally, listen to your body's signs and follow its

demands by prioritizing rest, relaxation, and rejuvenation. Get enough sleep, engage in things that bring you joy and fulfillment, and surround yourself with positive influences that elevate and motivate you on your quest.

**Stay Positive and Stay Persistent: You've Got This!**

Last, but not least, try to stay cheerful and stay consistent as you embark on your intermittent fasting experience. Rome wasn't built in a day, and neither is your journey to better health and well-being! Embrace the ups and downs, celebrate your accomplishments, and learn from your disappointments as you chart your course toward a better, happier you.

With a positive mindset and a persistent devotion to your goals, there's nothing you can't do with intermittent fasting by your side. So, gear up, buckle up, and get ready to go on the trip of a lifetime - your wellness journey awaits!

# Chapter 3

## Understanding Your Body's Needs

Welcome to Chapter 3, where we go on a quest to understand the mysteries of your body's demands and set the basis for a healthier, happier self. Get ready to roll up your sleeves, grab your magnifying glass, and unearth the clues that will unlock the secrets of good health and well-being!

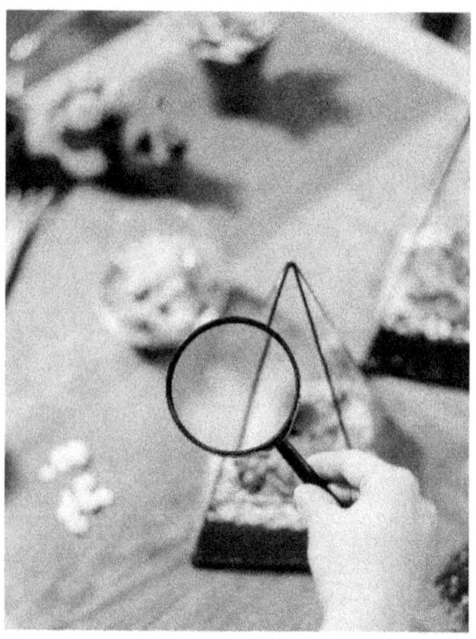

### Assessing Your Current Health and Lifestyle: The Detective's Toolkit

Imagine yourself as a detective, ready with a toolkit of questions, assessments, and observations to find the truth about your present health and lifestyle. Your purpose, should you choose to accept it, is to gather data, uncover patterns, and unearth insights that will guide you on your journey to wellness.

**Medical History:** Unraveling the Story of You First things first, let's start by diving into your medical history, the story of you documented in the pages of doctor's notes, lab reports, and prescription bottles. Take a journey down memory lane and reflect on your prior health experiences, from childhood illnesses to major surgeries, chronic ailments, and everything in between.

Understanding your medical history is like piecing together a puzzle, giving vital clues about your genetic predispositions, risk factors, and underlying health issues that may influence your present health status. So, take a pen and paper, scribble down any relevant information, and get ready to connect the dots!

**Lifestyle Factors:** The Habits That Make You Tick

Next up, let's throw a spotlight on your lifestyle determinants, the daily behaviors and routines that shape your health and well-being. Take time to focus on your food, exercise, sleep patterns, stress levels, and other lifestyle decisions that may affect your overall health and vitality.

Are you fueling your body with nutrient-rich foods that nourish and empower you? Or are you looking for sugary snacks and processed foods that leave you feeling sluggish and depleted? Are you emphasizing regular physical activity and mobility, or are you leading a sedentary lifestyle that's taking a toll on your health? These are just a few topics to consider when you examine your current lifestyle and discover areas for improvement.

**Environmental Influences:** Navigating Your Surroundings

In addition to your medical history and lifestyle considerations, it's crucial to examine the environmental effects that may affect your health and well-being. From air quality and water purity to exposure to poisons, pollutants, and electromagnetic radiation, your surroundings play a crucial impact in influencing your health results.

Take a moment to analyze your house, workplace, and other settings where you spend the majority of your time. Are there any potential hazards or health issues that you need to address? Are there actions you can take to create a healthier, more supportive atmosphere that promotes your well-being? By being attentive to your surroundings and making proactive efforts to eliminate dangers, you can create a healthier, happier living environment for yourself and your loved ones.

**Emotional and Mental Health**: Nurturing Your Inner Landscape

Last but certainly not least, let's not forget about your emotional and mental health, the inner landscape of ideas, feelings, and emotions that shape your total well-being. Take time to check in with yourself and reflect on your emotional condition, stress levels, coping techniques, and support systems.

Are you feeling overwhelmed and worn out by the demands of

daily life? Or are you experiencing emotions of melancholy, anxiety, or depression that may be harming your quality of life? It's vital to prioritize your emotional and mental health and seek support when required, whether it's through therapy, counseling, mindfulness practices, or simply reaching out to a trusted friend or loved one for support.

So there you have it, health detectives! By examining your current health and lifestyle, you're taking the first step towards understanding your body's demands and paving the way for a better, happier you. Armed with your detective's arsenal of questions, assessments, and observations, you're ready to unravel the secrets of your health and embark on the journey to wellness with confidence and determination.

## Identifying Dietary Needs and Restrictions: Nourishing Your Body from Within

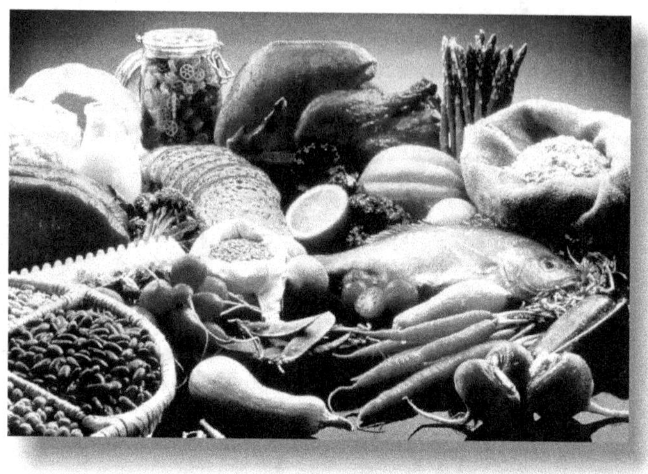

Now that we've built the basis by analyzing your medical history, lifestyle factors, environmental effects, and emotional well-being, it's time to shift our attention to one of the most critical areas of your health: your nutritional needs and constraints. Get ready to embark on a culinary adventure as we explore the intricacies of nourishing your body from within and providing it with the nutrition it needs to thrive!

Allergies and Sensitivities: Navigating the Culinary Minefield, First things first, let's start by identifying any allergies or sensitivities that may affect your nutritional choices. From familiar allergens like nuts, dairy, and shellfish to less obvious culprits like gluten, soy, and certain food additives, it's crucial to be aware of any potential triggers that may produce adverse reactions or discomfort.

Take time to think about any past experiences of allergic responses or sensitivities to certain foods, and consider speaking with a healthcare professional or allergist for testing if you suspect that you may have any underlying allergies or sensitivities. By being proactive and cautious about avoiding potential triggers, you can safeguard your health and well-being and enjoy a diet that's free from undesired side effects.

## Dietary Preferences and Restrictions: Honoring Your Body's Unique Needs

In addition to allergies and sensitivities, it's crucial to consider your dietary preferences and constraints when developing your nutrition plan. Whether you follow a specific diet like vegetarian, vegan, paleo, keto, or gluten-free, or you simply have personal preferences and tastes that dictate your food choices, it's crucial to acknowledge your body's unique needs and preferences.

Take some time to think about your dietary choices and constraints, and examine how they connect with your health and wellness goals. Are there any foods or food groups that you like to avoid or include in your diet? Are there any cultural or religious traditions that influence you're eating choices? By being attentive to your dietary preferences and constraints, you can build a nutrition plan that's personalized to your unique needs and interests.

## Nutritional Requirements: Meeting Your Body's Demands

Now let's speak about nutritional requirements, the building blocks of a balanced diet that give the key elements your body needs to perform efficiently. From macronutrients like carbohydrates, proteins, and fats to micronutrients like vitamins, minerals, and antioxidants, it's crucial to ensure that your diet is well-balanced and delivers all the nutrients your body needs to thrive.

Consider meeting with a licensed dietitian or nutritionist to examine your nutritional needs and design a personalized nutrition plan that suits your individual needs and goals. By focusing on nutrient-dense foods like fruits, vegetables, whole grains, lean meats, and healthy fats, you can fuel your body with the vitamins, minerals, and antioxidants it needs to maintain maximum health and well-being.

## Hydration: Quenching Your Body's Thirst

Last but certainly not least, let's not forget about hydration, the unsung hero of a balanced diet and lifestyle. Water is vital for practically every human function, from controlling body temperature and lubricating joints to assisting digestion and nutrition absorption. Yet many people fall short of reaching their daily hydration needs, resulting in dehydration and its related health hazards.

Make it a priority to stay hydrated throughout the day by drinking plenty of water and other hydrating beverages like herbal tea, coconut water, and infused water. Aim to drink at least eight glasses of water every day, and listen to your body's cues for thirst to ensure that you're staying appropriately hydrated. By emphasizing hydration, you can promote your overall health and well-being and ensure that your body gets the fluids it needs to perform efficiently.

So, there you have it, culinary explorers! By defining your dietary needs and constraints, you're taking a vital step towards nourishing your body from the inside and fueling it with the nutrition it needs to thrive. Whether you're navigating allergies and sensitivities, honoring your dietary preferences and constraints, achieving your nutritional requirements, or staying hydrated, you're on the way to maximum health and well-being. Bon appétit!

## Consulting with Healthcare Professionals: Your Trusted Partners in Health

As we venture deeper into the area of knowing your body's demands, it's crucial to acknowledge the invaluable role that healthcare experts play in guiding and supporting you on your path to well-being. Whether you're facing complex medical problems, managing chronic health difficulties, or simply seeking tailored counsel and advice, consulting with healthcare professionals can give you the experience, insight, and support you need to succeed.

### Primary Care Provider: Your First Line of Defense

Your primary care provider, whether it's a family physician, internist, or nurse practitioner, serves as your first line of defense in preserving and improving your overall health and well-being. Schedule regular check-ups with your primary care physician to review your baseline health status, track changes over time, and address any concerns or issues you may                                                            have.

During your sessions, be careful to address any medical history, lifestyle variables, environmental influences, or emotional and mental health difficulties that may impact your health and well-being. Your primary care provider can provide personalized counsel and recommendations tailored to your particular needs and goals, helping you negotiate the intricacies of your health with confidence and clarity.

## Registered Dietitian/Nutritionist: The Food Experts

When it comes to understanding the nuances of your dietary demands and constraints, a licensed dietitian or nutritionist can be your valued ally and guide. These food specialists are educated to assess your nutritional needs, establish tailored nutrition plans, and provide practical direction and support to help you accomplish your health and wellness objectives.

Consider scheduling a consultation with a licensed dietitian or nutritionist to examine your current food habits, identify areas for improvement, and build a nutrition plan that corresponds with your particular needs and preferences. Whether you're wanting to lose weight, manage chronic health issues, or maximize your general health and well-being, a licensed dietitian or nutritionist can give you the expertise and support you need to succeed.

## Allergist/Immunologist: Unraveling Allergy Mysteries

If you feel that you may have allergies or sensitivities to certain foods or environmental triggers, consultation with an allergist or immunologist can provide helpful insights and direction. These professionals are trained to diagnose and manage a wide range of allergic and immunological diseases, from food allergies and intolerances to environmental allergies and asthma.

Consider arranging allergy testing with an allergist or

immunologist to uncover any potential allergens or triggers that may be harming your health and well-being. Based on the results of your tests, your allergist or immunologist can provide individualized advice and treatment alternatives to help you manage your allergies and improve your quality of life.

## Mental Health Professional: Nurturing Your Emotional Well-Being

Last but certainly not least, don't neglect the importance of cultivating your emotional and mental well-being as part of your holistic approach to health and wellness. Consulting with a mental health expert, such as a psychologist, psychiatrist, therapist, or counselor, can provide vital support and guidance as you navigate the ups and downs of life.

Whether you're struggling with stress, anxiety, depression, grief, or other emotional or mental health difficulties, a mental health professional can provide a safe and supportive environment for you to explore your thoughts, feelings, and experiences. Through therapy, counseling, or other therapeutic interventions, you can build coping skills, resilience, and self-awareness to face life's problems with grace and perseverance.

By consulting with healthcare professionals, you're forming a trusted team of specialists to assist and support you on your journey to wellness. Whether you're seeking medical counsel, dietary assistance, allergy testing, or emotional support, your healthcare professionals are here to provide the expertise, insight, and support you need to succeed. Together, we'll manage the complexity of your health and enable you to live your greatest life!

# Chapter 4

# The Different Methods of Intermittent Fasting

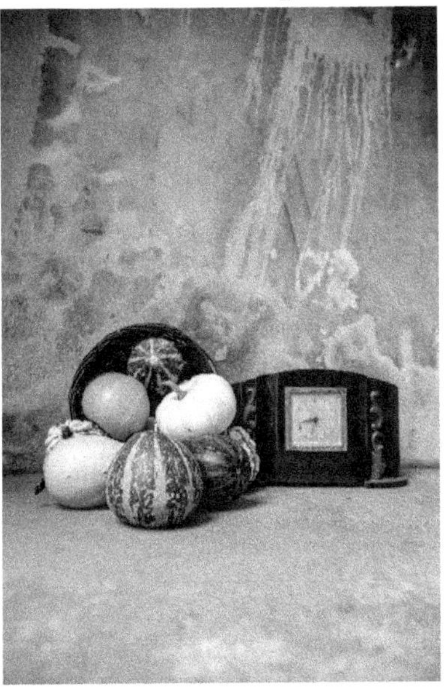

Welcome to Chapter 4, where we'll continue on a fascinating examination of the various approaches of intermittent fasting, each giving its own unique approach to harnessing the power of fasting for increased health and well-being. Get ready to explore the ins and outs of intermittent fasting and choose the strategy that's perfect for you!

## 16/8 Method: The Most Popular Fasting

# Protocol

Ah, the 16/8 technique - the superstar of the intermittent fasting world and possibly the most popular fasting protocol among novices and seasoned fasters alike. With its simplicity and flexibility, the 16/8 technique has grabbed the hearts and stomachs of health enthusiasts around the globe, giving a straightforward approach to intermittent fasting that's easy to implement and sustain.

So how does it work? Well, it's as straightforward as it sounds! With the 16/8 technique, you'll fast for 16 hours each day and restrict you're eating window to 8 hours, allowing your body to tap into stored fat for energy and gain a plethora of health benefits without feeling deprived or hungry.

**The Morning Sunrise to Evening Sunset Picture this:** you wake up in the morning, bask in the light of the dawn, and launch your day with a cool glass of water or a cup of black coffee to stave off hunger and rev up your metabolism. As the day develops, you go about your typical tasks, feeling motivated, focused, and ready to tackle whatever comes your way.

As the clock strikes noon, you break your fast with a nutritious and pleasant meal, nourishing your body with a balance of macronutrients and micronutrients to enhance your energy levels and overall well-being. From colorful salads to hearty soups to protein-packed stir-fries and grain bowls, the possibilities are unlimited!

**The Afternoon Delight and Evening Feast:** As the afternoon comes around, you have a light snack or two to keep hunger at bay and maintain your energy levels throughout the day. Whether it's a handful of nuts, a piece of fruit, or a tiny serving of yogurt, these mini-meals provide a welcome boost of nutrients and flavor to tide you over until dinner.

As the evening approaches, you settle down for a leisurely dinner with family or friends, relishing each bite and basking in the joy of shared meals and good company. From comfortable casseroles and substantial stews to fragrant curries and grilled delicacies, supper becomes a celebration of food, connection, and appreciation.

**The Sweet Taste of Success**

With the 16/8 approach, success tastes better than ever before! As you accept the simplicity and flexibility of intermittent fasting, you'll gain a plethora of health benefits, from improved metabolic health and weight management to enhanced cognitive performance and lifespan. Plus, with the option to tailor you're eating window to suit your lifestyle and interests, the 16/8 technique makes intermittent fasting feel like a breeze.

So go ahead, set your clock to the beat of the 16/8 method, and embark on the journey to better health and well-being with confidence and enthusiasm. With each passing day, you'll feel more empowered, more vibrant, and more alive than ever before, all thanks to the magic of intermittent fasting and the formidable 16/8 method!

The 16/8 technique is your passport to enhanced health, vigor, and well-being, delivering a straightforward and sustainable approach to intermittent fasting that's easy to adopt and enjoy. Whether you're a seasoned faster or a curious newbie, the 16/8 approach is sure to satisfy your taste senses and feed your body from the inside out. Here's to your health!

## 5:2 Method: Intermittent Calorie Restriction

Ah, the 5:2 Method - a blazing star in the constellation of intermittent fasting protocols, adored for its simplicity, flexibility, and tempting promise of increased health and life. With its roots in the concept of intermittent calorie restriction, the 5:2 Method offers a fresh approach to fasting that's as intriguing as it is successful.

So how does it work? Let's break it down! With the 5:2 Method, you'll alternate between two separate phases: five days of normal eating and two days of calorie restriction. During the five "feast" days, you'll enjoy your typical diet and eating habits, consuming a range of wonderful foods and flavors to your heart's content. But when the two "fast" days roll around, you'll restrict your calorie intake to a fraction of your typical diet, allowing your body to draw into stored fat for energy and gain a plethora of health benefits.

**Feast Days:** Indulge and Enjoy Welcome to the country of plenty, where feast days reign supreme and gourmet delights abound at every turn! During your five feast days, you'll bask in the joy of nourishing your body with a balance of macronutrients and micronutrients, savoring a range of great meals and flavors to boost your energy and satisfy your taste buds.

From vivid salads and substantial sandwiches to warm soups and indulgent desserts, the possibilities are unlimited on your feast days! Whether you're cooking up a storm in the kitchen or dining out at your favorite restaurant, feast days become a celebration of abundance, joy, and thankfulness for the healthy wealth that surrounds you.

**Fast Days:** Embrace the Challenge But wait, the adventure doesn't finish there! As the two fast days approach, you'll go on a journey of self-discovery and discipline, accepting the challenge of calorie restriction with courage and resolve. During your fast days, you'll consume a decreased number of calories, often about 500-600 for women and 600-700 for men, spread out over the course of the day.

While the concept of restricting calories may sound overwhelming at first, many fasters find that the experience is surprisingly easy, especially when armed with a few tactics and methods to make the most of their fasting days. From focusing on low-calorie, nutrient-dense foods like fruits, vegetables, lean proteins, and healthy fats to staying hydrated with plenty of water, herbal tea, and other calorie-free beverages, there are countless ways to navigate the challenges of calorie restriction and emerge victorious on your fasting days.

**The Sweet Taste of Success**

As you embrace the 5:2 Method and embark on the adventure of intermittent calorie restriction, you'll discover a renewed sense of empowerment, resilience, and vigor that transcends the bounds of time and location. With each passing day, you'll feel more energized, more focused, and more alive than ever before, all thanks to the magic of intermittent fasting and the magnificent 5:2 Method!

So there you have it, fasting trailblazers! The 5:2 Method is your passport to enhanced health, longevity, and well-being, giving a simple yet powerful method to intermittent fasting that's as effective as it is fun. Whether you're feasting on your favorite foods or embracing the challenge of calorie restriction, the 5:2 Method invites you to embark on a journey of self-discovery and transformation that's sure to satisfy your taste buds and nourish your body from the inside out. Here's to your health!

## Alternate Day Fasting and Extended Fasting

### Alternate Day Fasting

A dance of feast and famine, rhythm and regularity, as old as time itself. With its origins in ancient traditions and modern science, Alternate Day Fasting offers a unique method of intermittent fasting that's as intriguing as it is successful.

So how does it work? Let's plunge in! With Alternate Day Fasting, you'll alternate between fasting days and feast days, embracing a cycle of calorie restriction and normal eating that matches the ebb and flow of nature's rhythms. On fasting days, you'll consume minimum calories, often around 500-600 for women and 600-700 for males, whereas on feast days, you'll enjoy your usual food and eating habits without limitation.

**Fasting Days: Embrace the Challenge**

As the sun rises on your fasting days, you'll embrace the challenge of calorie restriction with courage and commitment. With each passing hour, you'll feel a sense of empowerment and resilience as you tap into your body's natural ability to burn stored fat for fuel.

While the concept of fasting may seem overwhelming at first, many fasters find that the experience is surprisingly manageable, especially when armed with a few tactics and strategies to make the most of their fasting days. From staying hydrated with plenty of water, herbal tea, and other calorie-free beverages to focusing on nutrient-dense foods like fruits, vegetables, lean proteins, and healthy fats, there are countless ways to navigate the challenges of calorie restriction and emerge victorious on your fasting days.

**Feast Days: Celebrate the Bounty**

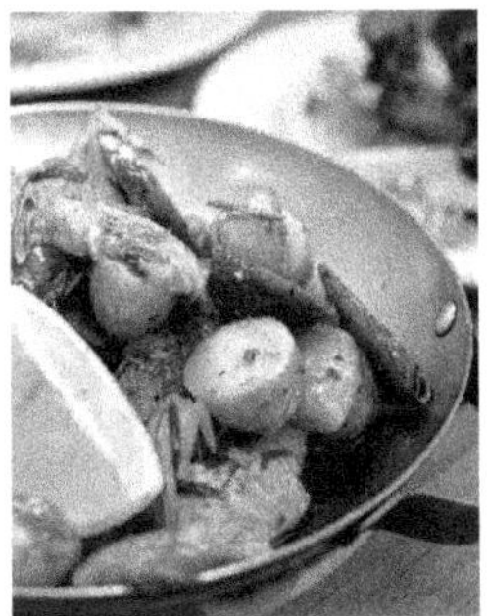

But fear not, for feast days are just around the way! As the fasting days draw to a close, you'll celebrate the abundance of nature's harvest and indulge in the pleasures of fueling your body with a range of delectable meals and flavors. From hearty meals and delectable sweets to refreshing snacks and tantalizing treats, feast days become a celebration of abundance, joy, and thankfulness for the healthy bounty that surrounds you.

Extended Fasting: Beyond the Limits

Now, let's change our focus to Extended Fasting - a voyage into the depths of fasting that stretches the bounds of time and place. With Extended Fasting, you'll start on a protracted fasting phase lasting anywhere from 24 hours to several days or even weeks, allowing your body to enter a state of profound ketosis and tap into its reservoirs of stored fat for energy. While the concept of Extended Fasting may sound scary at first, many fasters find that the practice is surprisingly fulfilling, giving a number of health benefits ranging from weight loss and improved metabolic health to enhanced cognitive function and longevity. Plus, with the supervision and support of healthcare professionals, fasting enthusiasts can safely negotiate the obstacles of Extended Fasting and emerge stronger, healthier, and more resilient than ever before.

So, there you have it, fasting explorers! Alternate Day Fasting and Extended Fasting offer unique ways of intermittent fasting that are as diverse as they are effective. Whether you're enjoying the cycle of feast and famine with alternate-day fasting or pushing the boundaries of time and place with Extended Fasting, your fasting journey awaits! So gear up, buckle up, and get ready to go on a voyage of self-discovery and transformation that's sure to please your senses and nourish your spirit.

# Chapter 5

# Meal Planning and Nutrition

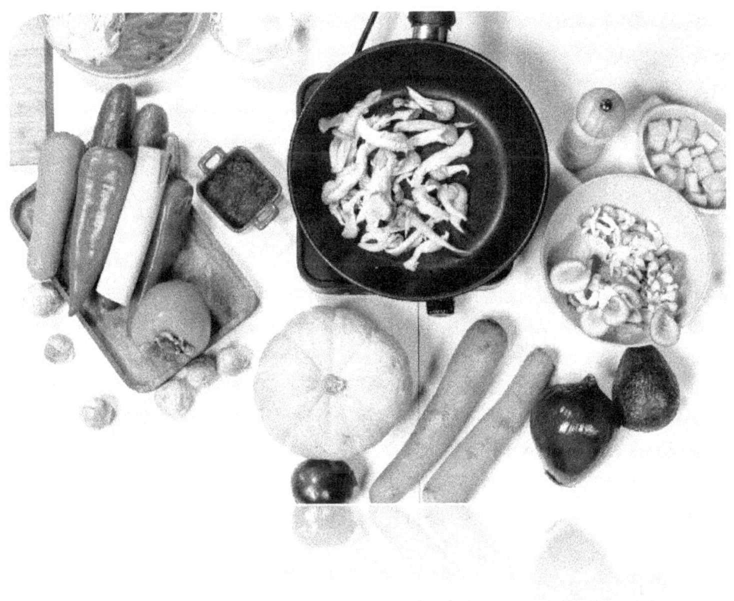

Welcome to Chapter 5, where we begin on a gastronomic voyage through the realm of meal planning and nutrition, revealing the secrets to crafting balanced meals that nourish and energize women over 50. Get ready to roll up your sleeves, polish your knives, and unleash your inner chef as we explore the art and science of producing tasty and nutritious meals that support your health and well-being!

## Designing Balanced Meals for Women Over 50: A Feast for the Senses

Ah, meal planning - the cornerstone of a healthy and vibrant existence, where imagination meets inspiration and flavor meets function in a beautiful dance of nourishment and delight. For women over 50, meal planning takes on new relevance, providing an opportunity to support hormonal shifts, metabolic needs, and overall well-being with every mouthful.

So how do we go about preparing balanced meals for ladies over 50? Let's break it down!

### Start with the Basics: Macronutrients and Micronutrients

First things first, let's start by understanding the building parts of a balanced meal: macronutrients and micronutrients. Macronutrients, including carbs, proteins, and fats, offer the energy your body needs to function efficiently, while micronutrients, such as vitamins, minerals, and antioxidants, support cellular health and immune function.

When preparing balanced meals, seek to incorporate a balance of macronutrients and micronutrients to promote your overall health and well-being. Incorporate a variety of colorful fruits and veggies, lean meats, whole grains, and healthy fats into your meals to ensure that you're getting a wide range of nutrients with every bite.

## Embrace the Power of Protein: The Building Blocks of Life

Next up, let's speak about the power of protein - the superhero of macronutrients that plays a critical role in supporting muscle growth and repair, hormone production, immunological function, and so much more. For women over 50, protein becomes especially crucial for sustaining bone health, muscular growth, and metabolic function as we age.

When planning your meals, make sure to incorporate a decent supply of protein with each meal, such as lean meats, chicken, fish, eggs, dairy products, tofu, tempeh, legumes, or plant-based protein sources like quinoa, lentils, and chickpeas. Aim to include roughly 20-30 grams of protein per meal to support your body's needs and keep you feeling satiated and energized throughout the day.

## Load Up on Colorful Fruits and Vegetables: Nature's Pharmacy

No balanced meal is complete without a hearty portion of colorful fruits and vegetables - nature's pharmacy of vitamins, minerals, and antioxidants that support immune function, heart health, brain function, and so much more. For women over 50, integrating plenty of fruits and vegetables into their meals becomes especially crucial for supporting bone health, cognitive function, and overall well-being.

When planning your meals, aim to fill half your plate with colored fruits and veggies to ensure that you're getting a wide range of nutrients with every bite. Choose a mix of colors and textures, from lush greens and vivid berries to crunchy carrots and sweet bell peppers, to create a feast for the senses that's as tasty as it is nutritious.

**Don't Forget the Healthy Fats: The Key to Satiety and Satisfaction**

Last but certainly not least, let's not forget about the necessity of healthy fats in a balanced meal. Contrary to common misconception, fats are not the enemy - in fact, they're vital for maintaining hormone synthesis, cognitive function, and nutritional absorption, as well as creating a sense of satiety and pleasure that keeps you feeling full and energized throughout the day.

When planning your meals, be sure to include a source of healthy fats, such as avocados, nuts, seeds, olive oil, fatty fish, or coconut oil, to give flavor, texture, and satiety to your meals. Aim to include a small serving of healthy fats with each meal to support your body's needs and keep you feeling satiated and energized throughout the day.

By constructing balanced meals that combine a balance of macronutrients and micronutrients, including plenty of protein, colorful fruits and vegetables, and healthy fats, you're setting yourself up for success on your journey to optimal health and well-being. So, grab your apron, sharpen your knives, and get ready to unleash your inner chef as you go on a culinary trip that's sure to thrill your taste senses and nourish your body from the inside out. Here's to your health!

## Foods to Emphasize and Avoid

### Foods to Emphasize: The Heroes of Your Plate

First, let's put a spotlight on the heroes of your plate - the tasty and nutritious foods that promote your health and well-being in more ways than one. From bright fruits and vegetables to lean meats, whole grains, and healthy fats, these foods provide the foundation of a balanced and satisfying diet that fuels your body with the nutrition it needs to thrive.

**Colorful Fruits and Veggies:** Load up on a rainbow of fruits and veggies to ensure that you're getting a diverse range of vitamins, minerals, and antioxidants with every bite. From lush greens and vivid berries to crunchy carrots and delicious bell peppers, these nutrient-packed foods boost immune function, heart health, cognitive function, and so much more.

**Lean Proteins:** Incorporate lean proteins into your meals to assist muscle growth and repair, hormone production, and immunological function. Choose from a variety of protein sources, including poultry, fish, eggs, tofu, tempeh, legumes, and plant-based protein sources like quinoa, lentils, and chickpeas, to add taste, texture, and fullness to your meals.

**Whole Grains:** opt for whole grains over refined grains to offer your body a continuous stream of energy and fiber that promotes digestive health and helps keep you feeling full and content. Choose whole grain options like brown rice, quinoa, barley, oats, and whole wheat bread, pasta, and crackers to add texture and taste to your meals.

**Healthy Fats:** Don't forget about the importance of healthy fats in your diet! Incorporate sources of healthy fats like avocados, nuts, seeds, olive oil, fatty fish, and coconut oil into your meals to support hormone production, brain function, and nutrient absorption, as well as provide a sense of satiety and satisfaction that keeps you feeling full and energized throughout the day.

Foods to Avoid: The Villains in Disguise

Next, let's talk about the villains in disguise - the meals that may harm your health and well-being if ingested in excess. From highly processed foods and sweet delights to harmful fats and refined carbs, these foods have little nutritional benefit and may lead to weight gain, inflammation, and chronic disease when taken consistently.

**Sugary goodies:** Beware of sugary goodies like candies, cookies, cakes, pastries, and sugary beverages, which supply empty calories and can wreak havoc on your blood sugar levels, energy levels, and waistline when taken in excess. Opt for naturally sweetened alternatives like fresh fruit, dried fruit, or modest amounts of dark chocolate to satisfy your sweet taste without the additional sugar.

**Highly Processed Foods:** Steer clear of highly processed foods like fast food, packaged snacks, frozen meals, and sugary cereals, which are often loaded with unhealthy fats, refined carbohydrates, artificial additives, and preservatives that offer little nutritional value and may contribute to inflammation, weight gain, and chronic disease over time.

**Harmful Fats:** Limit your intake of harmful fats like trans fats and saturated fats, which are found in fried foods, processed meats, butter, margarine, and high-fat dairy products. These fats can boost your cholesterol levels and increase your risk of heart disease when ingested in excess, so choose healthy alternatives like olive oil, avocado, nuts, seeds, and fatty seafood.

**Refined carbs:** Reduce your diet of refined carbs like white bread, white rice, white pasta, and sugary cereals, which are stripped of their fiber and nutrients during processing and can produce abrupt spikes and falls in blood sugar levels. Instead, consider whole grain products that give a consistent stream of energy and fiber to promote digestive health and keep you feeling full and content.

Nourish Your Body, Nourish Your Soul So there you have it, culinary adventurers! By emphasizing nutrient-dense meals like colorful fruits and vegetables, lean proteins, whole grains, and healthy fats, and avoiding processed foods, sugary snacks, unhealthy fats, and refined carbohydrates, you're feeding your body with the fuel it needs to thrive. So grab your apron, sharpen your knives, and get ready to go on a culinary trip that's sure to thrill your taste senses and nourish your body from the inside out. Here's to your health!

## Managing Nutrient Intake During Fasting Periods

Understanding Nutrient Intake During Fasting: A Balancing Act

Fasting periods can present a particular difficulty when it comes to maintaining appropriate food intake. While refraining from meals for extended periods offers a range of potential health benefits, it's crucial to ensure that your body obtains the essential nutrients it needs to sustain metabolic function, immunological health, and overall well-being.

During fasting periods, your body relies on stored foods to fuel key tasks and maintain metabolic balance. However, extended fasting can deplete key nutrients over time, potentially leading to vitamin shortages if not managed effectively. Therefore, it's vital to establish techniques to support nutritional intake during fasting periods and decrease the danger of deficiencies.

Strategies for Managing Nutrient Intake During Fasting:

**Prioritize Hydration:** Staying hydrated is crucial during fasting times to enhance cellular function, improve detoxification, and prevent dehydration. Aim to drink plenty of water throughout the day, and consider integrating electrolyte-rich liquids like herbal tea, bone broth, or electrolyte drinks to replenish lost minerals and support hydration.

**opt for Nutrient-Dense meals:** When breaking your fast, prioritize nutrient-dense meals that contain a diverse range of vitamins, minerals, and antioxidants to support general health and well-being. Focus on combining colorful fruits and veggies, lean meats, whole grains, and healthy fats into your meals to ensure that you're getting a balanced assortment of nutrients with every bite.

**Supplement Wisely:** In some situations, supplementation may be important to guarantee proper nutrient intake during fasting periods, especially if you're unable to satisfy your nutritional demands through diet alone. Consider introducing supplements like multivitamins, vitamin D, omega-3 fatty acids, and probiotics into your routine to cover any nutritional deficiencies and maintain optimal health.

**Practice attentive Eating:** When breaking your fast, practice attentive eating to boost nutrition absorption and optimize digestion. Chew your food slowly and completely, appreciating each bite and paying attention to hunger and satiety indicators. This thoughtful approach to eating can assist maximize nutrient intake and promote overall gut health during fasting periods.

**Monitor Your Health:** Finally, be sure to monitor your health attentively during fasting periods and speak with a healthcare expert if you have any indications or symptoms of vitamin deficiencies. Regular check-ups and blood tests can assist analyze your nutritional status and highlight any areas for improvement, allowing you to change your fasting routine and eating habits as needed to maintain optimal health and well-being.

By adopting ways to manage nutrient intake during fasting periods, you may guarantee that your body receives the critical elements it needs to flourish even when refraining from meals. From focusing on hydration and opting for nutrient-dense foods to supplementing appropriately and practicing mindful eating, there are various ways to promote good nutrition during fasting periods and maintain your health and well-being. Here's to fueling your body, even when fasting!

# Chapter 6

# Overcoming Challenges and Common Pitfalls

Welcome to Chapter 6, where we're going into the art of overcoming hurdles and managing frequent pitfalls on your intermittent fasting journey. In this chapter, we'll take a deep dive into the delicate world of managing hunger and cravings using a blend of medical expertise and practical techniques.

## Understanding Hunger: A Multifaceted Phenomenon

Hunger is a complex combination of physiological, psychological, and environmental elements that might impact our eating behavior. While it's typically considered a signal of physical need for nutrition, hunger can also be caused by emotional cues, contextual cues, and habitual patterns.

Physiologically, hunger is regulated by a complex network of hormones, including ghrelin (the hunger hormone), leptin (the satiety hormone), insulin, and glucagon, among others. These hormones act together to communicate with the brain and regulate hunger, energy balance, and metabolic function.

Psychologically, hunger can be impacted by factors such as stress, worry, boredom, and mood swings, which can create desires for specific foods or eating behaviors. Environmental signals, such as the sight or scent of food, social events, or time of day, can also promote hunger and impact our eating habits.

## Strategies for Managing Hunger and Cravings

Mindful Eating: Practice mindful eating by paying attention to your body's hunger and satiety indicators, as well as the sensory experience of eating. Take the time to take each bite, chew gently, and completely interact with the flavors, textures, and fragrances of your food. By listening to your body's cues and being present in the moment, you can boost your happiness and lessen the likelihood of overeating.

**Balanced Meals:** Design meals that are balanced in macronutrients (protein, carbs, and fats) to enhance satiety and stabilize blood sugar levels. Including protein-rich foods, fiber-rich carbohydrates, and healthy fats in your meals will help you feel full and content for longer durations, reducing the frequency and intensity of hunger and cravings.

**Hydration:** Stay hydrated throughout the day by drinking water, herbal tea, or other calorie-free liquids. Thirst can sometimes be confused for hunger, so being well-hydrated can help limit excessive nibbling or overeating. Aim to drink at least 8-10 glasses of water every day, and consider adding electrolytes or flavoring to boost taste and hydration.

**Strategic Snacking:** Incorporate nutritious snacks into your eating plan to help manage hunger between meals. Choose nutrient-dense foods like fruits, vegetables, nuts, seeds, yogurt, or whole-grain crackers to deliver continuous energy and keep cravings at bay. Be cautious of portion sizes and attempt to include a balance of carbohydrates, protein, and fats in your snacks to induce satiety.

**Distraction Techniques:** When cravings strike, distract yourself with activities that engage your mind and body, such as going for a walk, practicing yoga or meditation, or indulging in a pastime you enjoy. Redirecting your focus away from eating can help lower the intensity of cravings and boost your resilience to temptation.

**Emotional Support:** Seek emotional support from friends, family, or a support group to assist you in negotiating the hardships of fasting and retaining your dedication to your goals. Sharing your experiences, problems, and victories with others can provide support, accountability, and inspiration to keep on course.

As you continue on your fasting adventure, remember that regulating hunger and cravings is a skill that can be developed over time with practice, patience, and dedication. By recognizing the multidimensional nature of hunger, applying effective coping skills, and seeking support when needed, you may overcome hurdles and manage typical traps with confidence and grace.

So arm yourself with tenacity, resilience, and a dash of self-compassion as you embark on this revolutionary path to optimal health and well-being. Here's to embracing your inner resilience and defeating hunger and cravings one step at a time!

# Navigating Social Situations and Eating Out: The Art of Adaptation

Social gatherings, dining out with friends, and attending events are a vital part of our lives, providing opportunities for connection, celebration, and enjoyment. However, for persons practicing intermittent fasting, these situations might bring unique obstacles and temptations that may test their willpower and devotion to their fasting goals. Understanding the Challenges:

**Social Pressure:** In social settings, there may be pressure to conform to standard eating patterns or indulge in food and drinks that don't correspond with your fasting goals. Peer pressure, cultural standards, and societal expectations might impact your decisions and make it tough to keep to your fasting regimen.

**Limited Food Options:** Dining out at restaurants or attending activities may limit your access to fasting-friendly foods or make it harder to adhere to your desired eating schedule. Limited menu options, new products, and portion sizes might provide obstacles to keeping your fasting regimen and choosing healthier options.

**Mindless Eating:** In social circumstances, it's easy to engage in mindless eating or grazing on snacks and appetizers without paying attention to hunger cues or portion sizes. Buffet-style meals, sharing plates, and limitless food options can persuade you to overindulge and consume more calories than intended, leading to feelings of guilt or regret afterward.

## Strategies for Success:

**Plan Ahead**: Before attending social events or dining out, plan ahead by reading menus, researching restaurant selections, and conveying your dietary preferences or fasting intentions to your companions. Choose places that offer fasting-friendly options or customized meals that allow you to tailor your order to fit your needs.

**Be Flexible:** While it's crucial to stay devoted to your fasting regimen, it's equally essential to be flexible and adaptive in social circumstances. Recognize that some disruptions from your fasting schedule or meal plan are unavoidable and allow yourself some latitude to enjoy special events without shame or anxiety.

**Focus on Socializing:** Shift the focus of social gatherings away from food and drinks and toward meaningful connections and conversations with friends and loved ones. Engage in conversation, participate in activities, or propose alternative methods to bond that don't revolve around eating or drinking.

**Practice Moderation:** If presented with tempting food options or indulgent indulgences, practice moderation by opting for lesser portions, sharing dishes with others, or indulging in healthier alternatives when available. Allow yourself to enjoy your favorite foods in moderation while keeping careful of your overall calorie intake and nutritional balance.

**Stay Hydrated:** Keep hydrated at social events by drinking water, herbal tea, or other calorie-free liquids to help suppress appetite and prevent overeating. Sipping on a beverage can help keep your hands and mouth engaged, lessening the impulse to eat mindlessly.

**Be Assertive:** Don't be afraid to voice your dietary preferences or fasting goals nicely but strongly when faced with pressure to eat or drink in social settings. Advocate for yourself, convey your demands clearly, and don't feel pressured to justify or defend your choices to others.

Navigating social situations and dining out while practicing intermittent fasting involves a fine combination of preparation, flexibility, and boldness. By preparing ahead, being flexible, focusing on socializing, practicing moderation, being hydrated, and stating your requirements, you can continue your fasting schedule while still enjoying the company of friends and loved ones.

So embrace the social sides of life, relish the times of connection, and remember that intermittent fasting is about finding balance and harmony in both body and mind.

## Troubleshooting Plateaus and Setbacks: Strategies for Success

Plateaus and setbacks are a natural part of any journey toward health and fitness, including intermittent fasting. Whether you've struck a weight loss plateau, had a setback in your fasting regimen, or met problems that have disrupted your progress, it's crucial to approach these obstacles with perseverance, dedication, and a willingness to adapt.

## Understanding Plateaus

**Weight reduction Plateaus:** Plateaus in weight reduction occur when your body reaches a point of equilibrium, and progress pauses despite ongoing efforts to diet and exercise. Factors such as metabolic adaptability, hormonal oscillations, changes in exercise levels, and genetic predispositions can contribute to weight loss plateaus.

**Fasting Plateaus:** Fasting plateaus occur when your body adapts to your fasting practice, and progress slows or halts over time. Your metabolism may adjust to your eating schedule, and hormonal reactions may become less pronounced, leading to lessened impacts on weight loss, metabolic health, and other benefits associated with fasting.

## Strategies for Overcoming Plateaus and Setbacks:

**Review Your Progress:** Take a step back and review your progress objectively, evaluating factors such as changes in weight, body composition, energy levels, and overall well-being. Keep track of your fasting pattern, diet selections, exercise routine, and any other pertinent elements to find potential areas for improvement.

**Adjust Your Approach:** If you've hit a plateau or experienced a setback, consider modifying your approach to fasting, food, exercise, or lifestyle choices to restart progress and break through barriers. Experiment with different fasting protocols, meal times, calorie intake, macronutrient ratios, and exercise routines to determine what works best for your body.

**Emphasis on Non-Scale Victories:** Shift your emphasis away from the scale and celebrate non-weight victories such as increases in energy levels, mood, sleep quality, physical fitness, and overall well-being. Recognize that growth is not always linear and that tiny successes along the road are worth celebrating.

**Stay Consistent:** Maintain consistency with your fasting regimen, food, exercise, and lifestyle behaviors, even when progress seems slow or stagnant. Consistency is important to long-term success with intermittent fasting, and small, sustained adjustments over time can lead to considerable gains in health and well-being.

**Seek Support:** Reach out to friends, family, or a support group for encouragement, accountability, and motivation during hard times. Sharing your experiences, problems, and accomplishments with others can provide essential support and perspective, helping you stay on track with your fasting goals.

**Practice Self-Compassion:** Be kind to yourself and practice self-compassion throughout periods of plateaus and failures. Recognize that failures are a natural part of the journey toward health and well-being and that you're capable of overcoming problems with tenacity, determination, and self-care.

Plateaus and failures are unavoidable on the journey toward health and fitness, including intermittent fasting. By confronting challenges with tenacity, determination, and adaptation, you can overcome hurdles, break through barriers, and continue making progress toward your fasting goals. So embrace the adventure, learn from setbacks, and celebrate your perseverance as you manage the ups and downs of intermittent fasting with confidence and grace.

# Chapter 7

# Exercise and Physical Activity

Welcome to Chapter 7, where we'll continue our examination of the dynamic interaction between exercise and intermittent fasting. Prepare to go further into the realm of movement, sweat, and endorphins as we uncover the various advantages and tactics for incorporating exercise into your fasting regimen with extensive insights and a bit of fun!

## Maximizing the Benefits of Exercise During Fasting:

**Enhanced Weight Loss:** When paired with intermittent fasting, exercise becomes a potent tool for accelerating weight loss and encouraging fat loss. Fasting primes your body to burn stored fat for fuel, while exercise compounds this impact by increasing energy expenditure and metabolic rate. Whether you like cardio, strength training, or a combination of both, regular exercise can help you shed excess pounds and shape a leaner figure.

**Optimized Metabolic Health:** Intermittent fasting and exercise work synergistically to improve metabolic health indices such as insulin sensitivity, blood sugar control, and lipid profile. Fasting promotes insulin sensitivity, whereas exercise further enhances glucose absorption and use by skeletal muscles, reducing the incidence of insulin resistance and metabolic diseases including type 2 diabetes. Additionally, exercise produces positive changes in cholesterol levels, triglycerides, and blood pressure, further promoting cardiovascular health and general metabolic function.

**Increased Energy and Endurance:** Contrary to widespread assumption, exercising during fasting can actually boost energy levels and enhance physical performance. Fasted workouts tap into stored glycogen and fat stores for energy, resulting in sustained energy levels and better endurance during extended or high-intensity activity. Many individuals report feeling more awake, focused, and enthusiastic after fasted workouts, thanks to heightened levels of adrenaline and other stress hormones that enhance wakefulness and mental clarity.

**Muscle Preservation and Growth:** Intermittent fasting, when paired with resistance training, can help preserve lean muscle mass and increase muscle growth while promoting fat reduction. Fasting boosts the release of growth hormone, a crucial regulator of muscle development and repair, while exercise provides the stimulus needed to maintain muscle mass and stimulate protein synthesis. By including resistance training exercises like weightlifting, bodyweight workouts, or resistance bands in your fasting program, you can sculpt a stronger, leaner physique and avoid muscle loss over time.

**Mood Enhancement and Stress Reduction:** Exercise is a great mood enhancer and stress reducer, especially when undertaken during fasting. Physical activity boosts the release of endorphins, neurotransmitters that enhance emotions of happiness and well-being, while also reducing levels of stress hormones like cortisol. Fasting enhances these effects by boosting neuroplasticity and neuroprotection, resulting in better mood stability, resilience to stress, and overall mental well-being.

## Strategies for Success:

**Progressive Overload:** Incorporate progressive overload ideas into your training program to consistently test your muscles and drive growth. Gradually raise the intensity, duration, or volume of your workouts over time to avoid plateaus and maintain continual growth. Whether you're lifting heavier weights, increasing your training volume, or integrating more challenging activities, progressive overload is crucial to maximizing the benefits of exercise during fasting.

**Recovery and Regeneration:** Prioritize recovery and regeneration to support optimal muscle repair and growth between exercises. Adequate rest, sleep, hydration, and nutrition are crucial for refilling glycogen stores, rebuilding muscle tissue, and maximizing recovery after exercise. Consider combining active recovery exercises like stretching, foam rolling, yoga, or low-intensity cardio to boost circulation, minimize muscular soreness, and promote relaxation between intensive sessions.

**Periodization:** Implement periodization tactics to diversify your exercise program and prevent overtraining or burnout. Periodization entails separating your training program into several stages, each with its own specific goals, effort levels, and training modalities. By cycling between times of higher intensity, lower intensity, and recovery, you may enhance performance, prevent injuries, and sustain long-term adherence to your workout plan.

**Listen to Your Body:** Pay attention to your body's signals and alter your exercise program accordingly to avoid overtraining, injuries, or burnout. If you're feeling exhausted, sore, or mentally depleted, try taking a rest day or toning back the intensity of your workouts to allow for appropriate recovery. Remember that rest and recovery are just as vital as the exercise itself for getting optimal outcomes and avoiding setbacks.

**Enjoyment and diversity:** Find activities that you enjoy and include diversity in your fitness program to make things pleasant and engaging. Whether it's hiking, dancing, cycling, swimming, or playing sports, choose activities that offer you joy and correspond with your interests and preferences. Experiment with new training formats, surroundings, and social settings to keep your workouts fun and sustainable over the long run.

As you continue to embrace the synergy between exercise and intermittent fasting, remember that movement is not just a means to an end but a celebration of what your body is capable of doing. By adding regular exercise to your fasting program, you may maximize the benefits of both modalities and unlock your full potential for health, fitness, and vitality. So, lace up your sneakers, unleash your inner strength, and go on this amazing adventure toward a stronger, healthier, and happier self!

## Tailoring Workouts to Your Age and Fitness Level: A Personalized Approach

Exercise is a journey that evolves with time, impacted by elements such as age, fitness level, health state, and personal aspirations. Tailoring your workouts to correspond with your unique requirements and capabilities is vital for optimizing development, reducing injuries, and ensuring long-term adherence to your exercise regimen, especially within the context of intermittent fasting.

## Understanding Age-Related Considerations:

**Youth and Adolescence:** During youth and adolescence, the focus is frequently on creating a firm foundation of movement patterns, motor abilities, and cardiovascular health. Incorporating a variety of activities such as sports, games, and recreational play will assist build coordination, agility, and endurance while promoting a lifelong love of physical activity.

**Adulthood:** In adulthood, maintaining overall health, fitness, and functional capacity becomes a priority aim. Resistance training, cardiovascular exercise, and flexibility training are vital components of a well-rounded workout regimen, helping to sustain muscle mass, bone density, and mobility while supporting metabolic health and weight management.

**Middle Age:** As we enter middle age, the emphasis switches toward preventing age-related deterioration, controlling stress, and maintaining longevity. High-intensity interval training (HIIT), functional training, and mind-body activities like yoga and Pilates can help maintain cardiovascular health, muscle strength, and mental well-being while minimizing the risk of chronic diseases and cognitive decline.

**Older Adults:** In older adulthood, retaining independence, mobility, and quality of life becomes vital. Low-impact exercises, balance training, and resistance workouts utilizing small weights or resistance bands can assist enhance stability, reduce falls, and preserve functional capacity while limiting the risk of injury or joint strain.

## Strategies for Tailoring Workouts:

**Assess Your Fitness Level:** Start by measuring your current fitness level, including strength, endurance, flexibility, and mobility. Consider criteria such as your ability to perform fundamental movements, lift weights, complete aerobic activities, and recuperate from workouts. This self-assessment will help you identify areas of strength and weakness and customize your routines accordingly.

**Set Realistic Goals:** Establish realistic, achievable goals based on your age, fitness level, and personal preferences. Whether your goal is to gain muscle, increase cardiovascular fitness, lose weight, or enhance flexibility, defining clear, measurable, and attainable targets helps provide direction and incentive for your exercise regimen.

**Gradual Progression:** Progress gradually and steadily to minimize overexertion and reduce the chance of injury. Start with low-intensity activities and progressively increase the intensity, duration, or frequency of your workouts as your fitness level increases. Listen to your body and alter your workouts as needed to ensure that they stay demanding yet manageable.

**Modify Exercises:** Modify exercises to meet your unique needs and skills, especially if you have pre-existing health concerns or physical restrictions. For example, if you have joint discomfort or mobility concerns, you can perform seated or modified versions of exercises, use assistive equipment like resistance bands or stability balls, or focus on low-impact sports like swimming or cycling.

**Focus on Functional Fitness:** Prioritize exercises that increase functional fitness and address daily movement patterns and activities of daily living. Functional exercises like squats, lunges, push-ups, and planks assist in increasing strength, stability, and mobility in real-world settings, boosting your ability to do everyday chores with ease and confidence.

**Listen to Your Body:** Pay attention to your body's signals and alter your workouts accordingly to avoid overtraining, tiredness, or burnout. Rest when needed, prioritize sleep and recovery, and seek expert help if you feel persistent pain, discomfort, or trouble with particular exercises.

As you personalize your routines to your age and fitness level, remember that exercise is a lifelong journey that grows with you over time. By adopting a tailored strategy, setting reasonable objectives, moving gradually, changing exercises as needed, and listening to your body, you can enhance the efficiency of your workouts while fasting and empower yourself to reach your health and fitness goals at every stage of life.


# Maximizing the Benefits of Exercise and Fasting: Unleashing Synergy


Exercise and intermittent fasting are strong techniques for improving metabolic health, strengthening physical fitness, and promoting general well-being. When used effectively, these two techniques can synergistically magnify their effects, leading to higher fat loss, improved metabolic function, increased energy levels, and a multitude of other health benefits.


## Understanding the Synergy:

**Enhanced Fat Burning:** Fasting primes your body to burn stored fat for fuel, while exercise further amplifies this impact by raising energy expenditure and metabolic rate. When performed together, fasting and exercise create a synergistic environment that maximizes fat oxidation and accelerates weight loss, particularly when engaging in activities that stimulate both aerobic and anaerobic metabolism, such as high-intensity interval training (HIIT) or resistance training.

**Optimized Metabolic Health:** Both fasting and exercise independently improve metabolic health parameters such as insulin sensitivity, blood sugar control, and lipid profile. When combined, they synergistically augment these effects, leading to larger improvements in glucose management, lipid metabolism, and cardiovascular health. This synergy is particularly useful for people with insulin resistance, metabolic syndrome, or type 2 diabetes, as it can improve glycemic management, reduce insulin levels, and lessen the risk of cardiovascular problems.

**Increased Autophagy and Cellular Repair:** Fasting and exercise activate autophagy, a cellular mechanism that helps eliminate damaged or defective components, including proteins, organelles, and cellular detritus. Activating autophagy, fasting, and exercise synergistically increase cellular repair, rejuvenation, and regeneration, resulting in improved cellular function, longevity, and resistance to age-related illnesses.

**Elevated Mood and Cognitive Function:** Exercise boosts the production of endorphins, serotonin, and dopamine, neurotransmitters that promote emotions of euphoria, relaxation, and well-being. Fasting supports these effects by improving neuroplasticity, neurogenesis, and brain-derived neurotrophic factor (BDNF) levels, leading to increased emotional stability, cognitive function, and mental clarity. The synergistic combination of exercise and fasting can increase mood, reduce stress, and promote resilience against cognitive decline, benefiting both mental and emotional well-being.

## Strategies for Maximizing Benefits:

**Combine Different Modalities:** Incorporate a variety of cardiovascular activities, weight training, flexibility exercises, and mind-body practices into your fasting program to target different elements of fitness and maximize results.

Variety is crucial to minimizing plateaus, promoting general health, and keeping your workouts relevant and pleasant.

**Strategic scheduling:** Consider scheduling your workouts strategically to coincide with your fasting window for the best fat-burning and metabolic effects. Performing fasted exercises in the morning or before breaking your fast can boost fat oxidation and metabolic rate, while post-workout nourishment can help muscle recovery and repair.

**Hydration and Electrolytes:** Stay hydrated while fasting and exercising by drinking water, herbal tea, or other calorie-free beverages throughout the day. Electrolyte supplements may be advantageous, especially during lengthy or strenuous activities, to maintain electrolyte balance and prevent dehydration.

**Progressive Overload:** Gradually increase the intensity, duration, or frequency of your workouts over time to continue challenging your body and stimulate adaptability. Progressive overload is critical for increasing fitness gains, preventing plateaus, and obtaining long-term outcomes.

**Rest and Recovery:** Prioritize rest and recovery to allow your body to repair, rejuvenate, and adapt to the pressures of exercise and fasting. Adequate sleep, nutrition, and relaxation techniques are vital for maximizing recovery and decreasing the danger of overtraining, fatigue, or injury.

As you continue on your adventure of exercise and fasting, remember that the synergy between these two techniques can unlock a world of health, fitness, and energy. By deliberately combining fasting with exercise, you can maximize fat reduction, improve metabolic health, raise mood and cognitive function, and promote overall well-being. So embrace the power of synergy, unlock your potential, and go on this amazing adventure toward optimal health and vitality!

# Chapter 8

# Monitoring Progress and Adjusting Your Approach

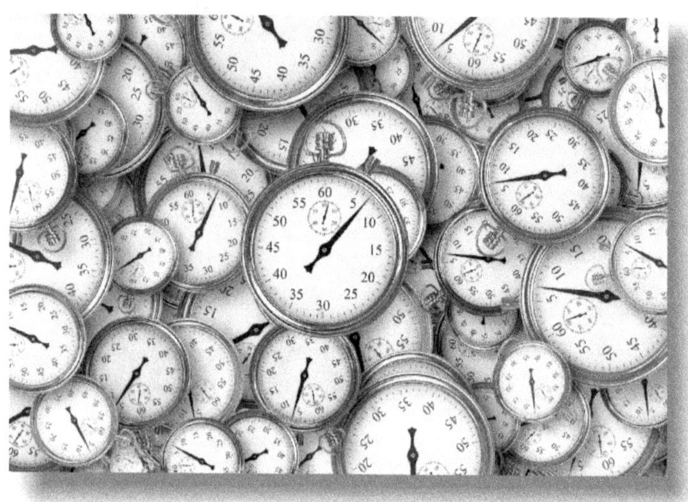

In this Chapter, we'll go on a voyage of self-discovery and optimization as we explore the crucial role of monitoring progress and altering your strategy within the area of intermittent fasting. Get ready to track your achievements, fine-tune your techniques, and unearth the secrets to long-term success with a dash of medical knowledge and a sprinkle of fun!

# Tracking Weight Loss, Energy Levels, and Other Metrics: The Path to Success

In the world of intermittent fasting, it isn't just about the numbers on the scale—it's about how you feel, how your body works, and how your general well-being grows over time. By tracking key metrics such as weight loss, energy levels, and other markers of health and vitality, you can obtain useful insights into your progress and make educated adjustments to your approach for optimal outcomes.

## Why Monitoring Progress Matters:

**Accountability and Motivation:** Tracking your progress provides a real measure of your successes and holds you accountable to your goals. Seeing positive changes in weight, energy levels, and other metrics can raise your motivation and strengthen your commitment to your fasting regimen, helping you stay on track even when faced with hurdles or setbacks.

**Identifying Patterns and Trends:** Monitoring progress allows you to identify patterns and trends over time, helping you understand how different aspects such as fasting protocols, dietary choices, exercise habits, and lifestyle behaviors affect your outcomes. By finding connections between particular activities and outcomes, you can make informed adjustments to enhance your strategy and maximize performance.

**Celebrating Milestones:** Tracking your progress helps you to celebrate milestones and victories along the way, no matter how minor or large. Whether it's completing a weight reduction goal, boosting energy levels, or witnessing changes in other health markers, celebrating your progress reinforces positive behaviors and encourages continuing effort and devotion.

**Course Correction:** Monitoring progress enables you to identify areas of improvement or areas where your strategy may need revision. Whether you're experiencing a plateau in weight loss, fluctuations in energy levels, or changes in other metrics, tracking allows you to course-correct and make targeted changes to your fasting schedule, diet, exercise, or lifestyle choices as needed.

## Key Metrics to Track:

**Weight Loss:** Keep track of changes in body weight over time to measure the effectiveness of your fasting program and food habits. While weight alone isn't the only measure of progress, it can provide significant feedback on the impact of fasting on fat loss and overall body composition.

**Energy Levels:** Monitor changes in energy levels, mood, and cognitive function throughout the day to measure the impact of fasting on your overall well-being. Notice any fluctuations in energy levels or changes in mental clarity, and identify probable factors that may be influencing your energy levels, such as hydration, sleep quality, or dietary choices.

**Hunger and Appetite:** Pay attention to hunger cues and appetite sensations during fasting periods to measure your body's response to your fasting routine. Notice any changes in hunger levels, cravings, or food choices, and alter your approach accordingly to better manage hunger and improve adherence to your fasting schedule.

**Physical Performance:** Track increases in physical performance, strength, endurance, and recovery to measure the influence of fasting on exercise performance and fitness gains. Notice any variations in workout intensity, duration, or recuperation time and alter your exercise regimen as needed to improve performance and prevent overtraining or injury.

**Biometric Markers:** Consider monitoring other biometric markers of health and vitality, such as blood pressure, blood sugar levels, cholesterol levels, and signs of inflammation or oxidative stress. These measures can provide additional insights into the influence of fasting on metabolic health, cardiovascular function, and overall well-being.

## Strategies for Tracking Progress:

Keep a notebook. Maintain a notebook or logbook to record daily or weekly observations, including changes in weight, energy levels, hunger, appetite, mood, physical performance, and other pertinent metrics. Use this notebook as a tool for self-reflection, goal setting, and course correction as you proceed on your fasting journey.

**Use Technology:** Take advantage of technology tools and programs designed to track health and fitness indicators, such as wearable fitness trackers, mobile apps, or internet platforms. These applications can automate the monitoring process, provide real-time feedback, and generate reports or visualizations to help you monitor progress and stay motivated.

**Schedule Regular Check-Ins:** Schedule regular check-ins with yourself to examine your progress, assess your goals, and make improvements to your strategy as needed. Set aside time each week or month to reflect on your path, acknowledge victories, and find areas for development or refinement.

**Seek Professional Help:** Consider obtaining help from healthcare specialists, nutritionists, or fitness trainers who may provide individualized recommendations and support based on your unique requirements and goals. Professional support can help you analyze your progress data, address any issues or challenges, and devise strategies for refining your fasting habits for long-term success.

As you embark on your journey of intermittent fasting, remember that improvement is a dynamic and evolving process that demands patience, perseverance, and self-awareness. By monitoring important variables like as weight loss, energy levels, hunger, appetite, and physical performance, you may obtain useful insights into your progress and make educated adjustments to your approach for optimal outcomes. So embrace the power of tracking, enjoy your victories, and continue to strive for health, vitality, and well-being as you journey toward a brighter, healthier future!

# Making Adjustments to Your Fasting Plan: The Path to Optimization

Intermittent fasting is not a one-size-fits-all method, and what works for one person may not necessarily work for another. As you go on your fasting journey, it's vital to be open-minded and willing to make alterations to your fasting strategy depending on your specific needs, preferences, and progress. By keeping flexible and adapting, you may modify your fasting practice to obtain optimal outcomes and long-term success.

## Why adjustments are necessary:

**Individual Variability:** Every individual is unique, with varying metabolic profiles, dietary preferences, lifestyle habits, and health considerations. What works for one person may not work for another, and it's crucial to acknowledge and respect these individual differences while planning and implementing a fasting plan.

**Changing Circumstances:** Life is dynamic, and circumstances may change over time, forcing alterations to your fasting plan. Factors such as job schedules, family responsibilities, vacation plans, social engagements, and seasonal changes can all affect your ability to adhere to a rigid fasting schedule and may necessitate flexibility in your approach.

**Proceed and Plateau:** As you proceed on your fasting journey, you may encounter variations in weight, energy levels, hunger, and other metrics that need adjustments to your fasting schedule. Plateaus pauses, or swings in progress are common occurrences and may suggest the need for alterations to your fasting procedure, dietary habits, exercise program, or lifestyle choices.

**Health Considerations:** Your health state, medical history, and dietary demands may alter over time, forcing revisions to your fasting plan to fit changing circumstances or health considerations. Certain medical problems, medications, or dietary restrictions may require modifications to your fasting protocol under the advice of healthcare professionals.

## Strategies for Making Adjustments:

**Listen to your body:** Pay attention to your body's signals and feedback, including hunger cues, energy levels, mood, digestion, and overall well-being. If you're feeling unusually weary, angry, or hungry during fasting times, it may be a sign that your fasting strategy is too rigid or unsustainable and may require change.

**Experiment and iterate:** Take a flexible and experimental attitude to fasting and be willing to test different fasting protocols, durations, and techniques to determine what works best for you. Experiment with alternatives such as alternate-day fasting, time-restricted eating, or modified fasting schedules to find the strategy that corresponds with your goals, preferences, and lifestyle.

**Gradual modifications:** Implement modifications to your fasting strategy gradually and progressively to enable your body to adapt and adjust. Whether you're increasing fasting durations, modifying feeding windows, or implementing new dietary or lifestyle habits, incremental modifications are more sustainable and simpler to adhere to over the long run.

**Measure and assess:** Continuously evaluate your progress, measure key indicators, and assess the impact of alterations to your fasting strategy on your health, fitness, and well-being. Keep a notebook or logbook to record observations, track changes in weight, energy levels, hunger, mood, and other important characteristics, and use this data to inform future adjustments.

**Seek Guidance:** Consult with healthcare specialists, dietitians, or fasting experts if you're unclear about how to adapt your fasting strategy or if you have unique health issues or considerations. Professional advice can provide individualized recommendations, address any issues or challenges, and ensure that alterations to your fasting plan are safe, successful, and tailored to your individual needs.

## Common Adjustments to Consider:

**Modifying Fasting Duration:** Adjust the duration of your fasting times to better correspond with your lifestyle, schedule, and metabolic needs. Whether you're shortening or prolonging fasting durations, experimenting with different fasting protocols, or introducing fasting modifications, find the technique that best meets your goals and interests.

**Adjusting food Windows:** Modify the timing and duration of your food windows to optimize nutritional intake, support energy levels, and promote satiety. Whether you're modifying meal schedules, frequency, or composition, prioritize nutrient-dense meals, balanced macronutrient ratios, and mindful eating behaviors to support general health and well-being.

**Fine-Tuning Meal Composition:** Fine-tune the composition of your meals to ensure optimal nutrient intake, increase metabolic flexibility, and support your fasting goals. Whether you're modifying macronutrient ratios, portion sizes, or dietary choices, focus on whole, minimally processed foods and prioritize nutrient-rich sources of protein, healthy fats, fiber, vitamins, and minerals.

**Optimizing Exercise Routine:** Evaluate your exercise routine and consider making alterations to better align with your fasting plan, goals, and preferences. Whether you're modifying workout time, intensity, duration, or frequency, prioritize activities that support your goals, increase metabolic health, and promote overall fitness and well-being.

As you navigate your fasting path, remember that flexibility and adaptation are crucial to long-term success. By keeping open-minded, listening to your body, trying new ways, and making educated adjustments as needed, you may improve your fasting strategy to achieve optimal results and sustain your success over the long run. So enjoy the trip, trust the process, and remain devoted to self-discovery and optimization as you continue to harness the transforming power of intermittent fasting!

## Celebrating Milestones and Staying Motivated: Fueling Your Fasting Journey

Intermittent fasting is a journey filled with obstacles, wins, and breakthroughs, and celebrating milestones along the way is vital for sustaining momentum and keeping motivated.

Whether it's meeting a weight reduction goal, boosting energy levels, or learning a new fasting protocol, taking the time to appreciate and celebrate your achievements may fuel your enthusiasm and motivate continued growth.

## Why Celebrating Milestones Matters:

**Positive Reinforcement:** Celebrating milestones gives positive reinforcement for your efforts and achievements, encouraging the behaviors and habits that lead to your success. Recognizing progress and celebrating victories can enhance your confidence, self-esteem, and belief in your capacity to reach your goals, inspiring you to persevere through challenges and failures.

**Emotional Well-Being:** Celebrating milestones boosts your emotional well-being and sense of fulfillment, creating a good attitude and approach toward your fasting journey. By focusing on the progress you've made and the goals you've achieved, you build a sense of thankfulness, fulfillment, and joy that uplifts your spirits and energizes your dedication to continued growth and improvement.

**Maintaining Momentum:** Celebrating milestones helps you retain momentum on your fasting journey, preventing fatigue, boredom, or complacency. By reducing your path into smaller, attainable milestones and enjoying each step along the way, you build a sense of progress and forward momentum that propels you toward your ultimate goals.

**Building Resilience:** Celebrating milestones increases resilience and fortitude, helping you overcome setbacks, hurdles, or problems that may happen along the path. By focusing on your achievements and the progress you've made, you create a sense of resilience, tenacity, and perseverance that encourages you to overcome adversity and keep pushing forward in the face of hurdles.

## Strategies for Celebrating Milestones:

**Set clear goals:** Establish clear, detailed, and achievable goals that act as milestones on your fasting journey. Whether it's losing a specific amount of weight, finishing a fasting challenge, or boosting energy levels, make goals that are meaningful, measurable, and motivating to you.

**Track Your Progress:** Monitor your progress and track key indicators to quantify your achievement and celebrate milestones along the way. Keep a notebook, logbook, or progress tracker to record your achievements, measure changes in weight, energy levels, and other pertinent aspects, and celebrate each milestone as you reach it.

**Praise Yourself:** Reward yourself for hitting milestones and achieving goals, whether it's treating yourself to a healthy meal, indulging in a favorite pastime, or purchasing a modest prize as a token of your accomplishment. Choose prizes that correspond with your aims and values and serve as positive reinforcement for your achievements.

**Share Your Achievements:** Share your achievements and milestones with others, whether it's friends, family, or members of your fasting community. Celebrate your victories openly, post your progress on social media, or join online forums or support groups where you may interact with others who are on a similar road and celebrate milestones together.

**Reflect and Appreciate:** Take time to reflect on your achievements and appreciate the progress you've made on your fasting journey. Practice appreciation for the changes you've encountered, the lessons you've learned, and the progress you've gained along the road, and celebrate the journey as much as the goal.

## Staying Motivated:

**Visualize Success:** Visualize your goals and success regularly, imagining yourself attaining your desired outcomes and feeling the rewards of your fasting journey. Visualization techniques can assist in reinforcing your motivation, focus your efforts, and keep you inspired and determined to attain your goals.

**Stay Inspired:** Seek inspiration from those who have achieved similar goals or overcome comparable hurdles on their fasting journey. Follow success stories, read books, watch documentaries, or listen to podcasts that inspire and motivate you to be committed to your fasting objectives and aspirations.

**Find Joy in the Journey:** Find joy in the journey and embrace the process of self-discovery, growth, and transformation that accompanies your fasting journey. Focus on the positive aspects of your experience, celebrate minor triumphs, and face problems with a spirit of curiosity, resilience, and optimism.

**Connect with Support:** Connect with a supportive community of like-minded individuals who can offer encouragement, guidance, and accountability on your fasting journey. Whether it's joining online forums, attending local gatherings, or engaging in group challenges, surround yourself with a supportive network that uplifts and pushes you to stay committed to your goals.

**Practice self-care:** prioritize self-care and well-being to preserve balance and resilience on your fasting journey. Take time to rest, recharge, and nourish yourself physically, intellectually, and emotionally, embracing activities such as meditation, mindfulness, relaxation techniques, or hobbies that offer you joy and fulfillment.

 As you navigate your fasting journey, remember to enjoy each milestone along the way, no matter how minor or large. By celebrating your achievements, creating new goals, and keeping inspired, you may fuel your passion and desire to continue working toward your ultimate health and wellness dreams. So embrace the adventure, appreciate your victories, and stay encouraged as you embark on this revolutionary route toward a greater, healthier future!

# Chapter 9

# Intermittent Fasting and Long-Term Health

Welcome to Chapter 9, where we'll go on a fascinating journey into the world of intermittent fasting and its tremendous impact on long-term health. In this episode, we'll dig beyond weight reduction and find the variety of other health benefits that intermittent fasting offers, all while maintaining a vibrant and engaging tone.

## Beyond Weight Loss: Other Health Benefits of Intermittent Fasting

Intermittent fasting isn't just about dropping pounds it's a holistic approach to health and wellness that delivers a myriad of benefits beyond the scale. From increasing metabolic function to encouraging cellular repair and longevity, intermittent fasting can change your health and vitality in ways that reach far beyond weight loss alone.

Exploring the Multifaceted Benefits:

**Improved Metabolic Health:** Intermittent fasting has been proven to improve numerous indices of metabolic health, including insulin sensitivity, blood sugar control, and lipid profile. By boosting metabolic flexibility and reducing insulin resistance, intermittent fasting may lessen the risk of type 2 diabetes, metabolic syndrome, and cardiovascular disease, leading to enhanced overall health and longevity.

**Enhanced Cellular Repair:** Fasting activates a process called autophagy, where cells break down and recycle damaged or defective components, enabling cellular repair, regeneration, and rejuvenation. By boosting autophagy, intermittent fasting may support healthy aging, minimize the risk of age-related illnesses, and enhance cellular resilience and longevity.

**Reduced Inflammation: Chronic** inflammation is a critical driver of many chronic diseases, including heart disease, cancer, and neurological disorders. Intermittent fasting has been proven to reduce inflammation levels in the body, potentially lowering the risk of inflammatory disorders and boosting overall health and well-being.

**Brain Health and Cognitive Function:** Intermittent fasting has neuroprotective effects and may improve brain health and cognitive function. By boosting the generation of brain-derived neurotrophic factor (BDNF) and encouraging neurogenesis, intermittent fasting may enhance learning, memory, and cognitive function while reducing the risk of neurodegenerative illnesses such as Alzheimer's and Parkinson's.

**Longevity and Aging:** Emerging evidence suggests that intermittent fasting may increase lifespan and promote healthy aging by activating longevity pathways such as AMPK and SIRT1. By boosting cellular stress tolerance, DNA repair mechanisms, and mitochondrial function, intermittent fasting may reduce the aging process and enhance the lifespan of numerous creatures, including humans.

**Embracing the Journey to Long-Term Health**

**Educate yourself:** Take the time to educate yourself about the science behind intermittent fasting and its possible health advantages. Understanding how fasting affects your body at a molecular level will enable you to make informed decisions and embrace the fasting journey with confidence and passion.

**Start Slow:** If you're new to intermittent fasting, start slow and gradually ease into your fasting regimen. Begin with shorter fasting periods or less stringent fasting protocols, and gradually increase the time or intensity as your body adapts and you become more comfortable with fasting.

**Stay Consistent:** Consistency is crucial to obtaining the long-term benefits of intermittent fasting. Stick to your fasting plan, especially on days when it feels tough, and trust the process. Over time, your body will adjust to the fasting pattern, and you'll begin to experience the transforming impacts of fasting on your health and well-being.

**Listen to Your Body:** Pay attention to your body's signals and adapt your fasting schedule as needed based on how you feel. If you develop chronic fatigue, dizziness, or other unpleasant effects, consider changing your fasting strategy or obtaining help from a healthcare practitioner.

**Focus on Whole Foods:** opt for nutrient-dense, whole foods during your eating window to support general health and well-being. Prioritize fresh fruits, vegetables, lean proteins, healthy fats, and whole grains, and eliminate processed foods, sugary snacks, and refined carbohydrates.

As you embark on your adventure of intermittent fasting, realize that the benefits extend far beyond weight reduction alone. By embracing the many benefits of intermittent fasting, including increased metabolic health, enhanced cellular repair, reduced inflammation, brain health, and longevity, you may transform your health and vitality and embrace a vibrant, meaningful life for years to come. So embrace the journey, enjoy your health, and uncover the transformative power of intermittent fasting for long-term health and well-being!

## Lowering the Risk of Age-Related Diseases: Unveiling the Science

As we age, the risk of developing chronic diseases such as heart disease, cancer, diabetes, and neurological disorders increases. However, increasing research suggests that intermittent fasting may offer a robust defense against age-related diseases, helping to minimize their start and progression by targeting fundamental underlying mechanisms of aging and disease development.

### Understanding the Mechanisms:

**Reduced Inflammation:** Chronic inflammation is a hallmark of many age-related disorders and contributes to their development and progression. Intermittent fasting has been found to reduce inflammation levels in the body, suppressing the inflammatory response and lowering the risk of illnesses such as heart disease, arthritis, and Alzheimer's disease.

**Improved Metabolic Health:** Age-related alterations in metabolism, including insulin resistance, dyslipidemia, and decreased glucose tolerance, have a key role in the development of diabetes, obesity, and cardiovascular disease. Intermittent fasting promotes metabolic health by boosting insulin sensitivity, promoting fat loss, and reducing blood sugar and cholesterol levels, therefore minimizing the risk of metabolic illnesses and their associated problems.

**Enhanced Cellular Repair:** As we age, cellular repair systems become less efficient, resulting in the accumulation of damaged or defective components within cells. Intermittent fasting activates autophagy, a cellular mechanism that clears away damaged organelles and proteins, improving cellular repair, rejuvenation, and resilience against age-related damage and disease.

**Increased Stress Resistance:** Intermittent fasting stimulates stress response pathways such as AMPK and sirtuins, which boost cellular stress resistance and prolong lifespan. By activating these pathways, intermittent fasting may boost cellular resilience to environmental stressors, oxidative damage, and other age-related insults, thereby lowering the risk of age-related illnesses and extending lifespan.

Practical Strategies for Harnessing the Benefits:

**Adopting a Consistent Fasting Routine:** Consistency is crucial to reaping the long-term advantages of intermittent fasting for reducing the risk of age-related illnesses. Establish a regular fasting schedule that corresponds with your lifestyle and tastes, and stick to it consistently to maximize its effectiveness in promoting good aging and lifespan.

**Balancing Nutrient Intake:** While fasting, it's crucial to maintain enough nutrient intake to support general health and well-being. Focus on nutrient-dense, whole foods throughout your eating windows, including fruits, vegetables, lean proteins, healthy fats, and whole grains, and minimize processed foods, sugary snacks, and refined carbohydrates.

**Incorporating Physical Activity:** Regular physical activity is vital for supporting healthy aging and reducing the risk of age-related disorders. Incorporate a combination of aerobic activity, strength training, flexibility exercises, and balance activities into your regimen to enhance cardiovascular health, muscle strength, bone density, and overall mobility.

**Managing Stress:** Chronic stress accelerates the aging process and raises the risk of age-related disorders. Practice stress management practices such as mindfulness meditation, deep breathing exercises, yoga, tai chi, or progressive muscle relaxation to lower stress levels and increase emotional well-being and resilience.

**Prioritizing Sleep:** Adequate sleep is vital for maintaining optimal health and minimizing the risk of age-related disorders. Aim for seven to nine hours of quality sleep every night, and prioritize sleep hygiene measures such as maintaining a regular sleep schedule, setting a calming bedtime routine, and optimizing your sleep environment for restorative sleep.

As we journey through life, it's crucial to focus on our health and well-being to promote healthy aging and lower the risk of age-related disorders. By embracing the potential benefits of intermittent fasting, including lower inflammation, improved metabolic health, greater cellular repair, and increased stress tolerance, we can empower ourselves to age gracefully, preserve vitality, and have a bright, satisfying life for years to come. So, embrace the power of intermittent fasting, adopt good living choices, and embark on the journey toward healthy aging and longevity with confidence and joy!

## Maintaining a Healthy Lifestyle Beyond Fasting: A Holistic Approach

While intermittent fasting offers several health benefits, maintaining a healthy lifestyle goes beyond fasting alone. By adopting a holistic strategy that incorporates nutrition, physical exercise, stress management, sleep hygiene, and other lifestyle aspects, you can enhance your health and well-being for the long term, complementing the benefits of intermittent fasting and increasing overall vitality.

Key Components of a Healthy Lifestyle:

**Nutrition:** Optimal nutrition is the foundation of a healthy lifestyle, supplying critical nutrients that promote cellular function, metabolism, and overall well-being. Focus on having a balanced diet rich in fruits, vegetables, whole grains, lean proteins, and healthy fats, and minimize intake of processed foods, sugary snacks, and refined carbohydrates.

**Physical Activity:** Regular physical activity is vital for maintaining cardiovascular health, muscle strength, bone density, and overall mobility. Incorporate a range of activities into your regimen, including aerobic activity, strength training, flexibility exercises, and balancing activities, and aim for at least 150 minutes of moderate-intensity exercise per week.

**Stress Management:** Chronic stress can significantly impact health and well-being, contributing to inflammation, hormone imbalances, and other undesirable impacts. Practice stress management strategies such as mindfulness meditation, deep breathing exercises, yoga, tai chi, or progressive muscle relaxation to lower stress levels and build emotional resilience.

**Sleep hygiene:** adequate sleep is vital for sustaining cognitive function, mood control, immunological function, and overall health. Prioritize healthy sleep hygiene habits such as maintaining a regular sleep schedule, setting a peaceful evening routine, optimizing your sleep environment, and avoiding stimulants such as caffeine and electronics before bedtime.

**Hydration:** Staying hydrated is vital for maintaining optimal hydration levels, supporting digestion, circulation, temperature regulation, and overall health. Aim to drink lots of water throughout the day, and consider integrating hydrating items such as fruits, vegetables, and herbal teas into your diet to maintain hydration.

## Integration with Intermittent Fasting:

**Balanced Nutrition:** While fasting, prioritize nutrient-dense, whole meals throughout your eating windows to enhance general health and well-being. Ensure enough intake of important nutrients such as vitamins, minerals, protein, and fiber, and avoid excessive consumption of processed foods, sugary snacks, and refined carbohydrates.

**Physical Activity:** Incorporate physical activity into your fasting practice to boost cardiovascular health, muscle strength, and general fitness. Schedule workouts during your eating windows or opt for low-intensity activities such as walking or yoga during fasting periods to support energy levels and metabolism.

**Stress Management:** Practice stress management strategies such as mindfulness meditation, deep breathing exercises, or progressive muscle relaxation during fasting periods to lower stress levels and increase emotional well-being. Engage in activities that encourage relaxation and renewal, such as reading, listening to music, or spending time in nature.

**Sleep Quality:** Prioritize appropriate sleep hygiene habits to promote sleep quality and duration during fasting periods. Establish a consistent sleep schedule, build a peaceful nighttime routine, and avoid interruptions to your sleep environment to support restorative sleep and overall well-being.

**Hydration:** Stay hydrated during fasting periods by drinking plenty of water and including hydrating items such as fruits, vegetables, and herbal teas into your diet. Monitor your hydration levels and heed your body's signals to ensure appropriate hydration throughout the day.

As you embrace intermittent fasting as a valuable strategy for enhancing long-term health and energy, remember that sustaining a healthy lifestyle extends beyond fasting alone. By incorporating diet, physical exercise, stress management, sleep hygiene, and hydration into your daily routine, you may enhance your health and well-being, complementing the benefits of fasting and maintaining overall vitality for years to come.

So, embrace the holistic approach to health and wellness, prioritize self-care, and embark on the journey toward optimal health and vitality with confidence and joy!

# Chapter 10

# Final Thoughts and Conclusion

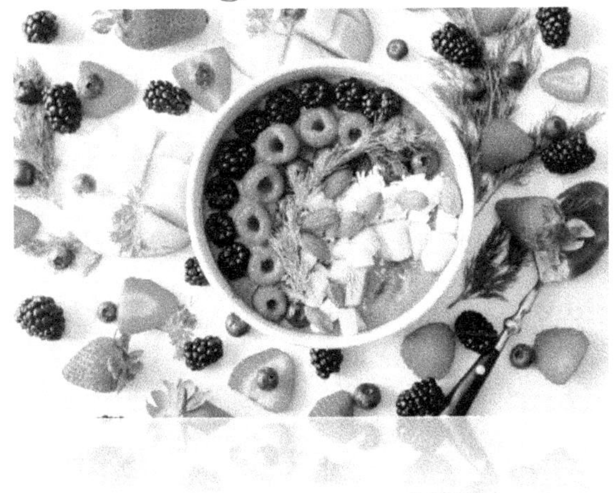

Welcome to the final chapter of your intermittent fasting journey, a time to reflect, enjoy, and embrace the significant changes you've experienced along the road. In this segment, we'll take a minute to look back on your accomplishments, appreciate the lessons learned, and set the stage for a vibrant, healthy future filled with vitality and well-being.

* * *

# Reflecting on Your Intermittent Fasting Journey: A Transformative Experience

As you stand at the climax of your intermittent fasting adventure, take a moment to pause and reflect on the remarkable transformations you've undergone both inside and out. From reducing unwanted pounds to boosting energy levels, expanding mental clarity, and improving general health, your journey has been nothing short of incredible.

**Celebrating Your Achievements:** **Weight Loss:** Whether you embarked on this road to reduce excess weight or not, chances are you've experienced major changes in your body composition. Celebrate your victories, no matter how big or small, and take satisfaction in the progress you've made toward a better, happier you. Energy and vibrancy: Notice how your energy levels have skyrocketed throughout your fasting journey, providing you with the vibrancy and enthusiasm for life you may not have felt in years. Revel in the fresh sensation of vigor and enthusiasm that accompanies your revived body and mind.

**Mental Clarity:** Embrace the mental clarity and sharpness of mind that intermittent fasting has placed upon you, helping you to handle problems with confidence and focus. Take joy in the higher cognitive function and greater memory that has become your new norm.

**Health Improvements:** Consider the plethora of health benefits you've encountered along the journey, from improved metabolic health and lower inflammation to greater cellular repair and resilience. Applaud yourself for making proactive efforts toward a better, more vibrant future.



**Tenacity:** Through the ups and downs of your fasting adventure, you've exhibited incredible tenacity and determination. Embrace the hardships you've experienced as chances for growth and learning, knowing that each obstacle has strengthened your resolve and moved you forward.

**Self-Discovery:** Alongside your physical transformations, you've gone on a journey of self-discovery and empowerment. Embrace the heightened sense of self-awareness and confidence that comes with taking ownership of your health and well-being.

**Adaptability:** Throughout your intermittent fasting experience, you've learned to adapt and evolve, adapting your strategy as needed to meet your changing requirements and circumstances. Celebrate your adaptability and readiness to tackle new challenges with an open mind and a bold attitude.

**Mindfulness:** In the hustle and bustle of daily life, intermittent fasting has given you an opportunity to build mindfulness and presence. Cherish the times of stillness and reflection that fasting has offered you, allowing you to reconnect with yourself and the world around you. Looking Ahead: A Bright and Healthy Future

As you bid farewell to this chapter of your intermittent fasting journey, know that the road ahead is filled with unlimited possibilities for development, vigor, and well-being. Armed with the information, experience, and resilience gathered along the road, you're set to embrace a future bursting with health, happiness, and fulfillment.

Final        Words        of        Encouragement:

**Stay Curious:** Approach each day with a sense of curiosity and amazement, embracing new challenges and possibilities for growth with an open heart and an adventurous spirit. Keep Moving Forward: No matter where your journey leads you, remember that progress is never linear. Embrace the highs and lows with grace and resilience, knowing that each stride forward puts you closer to your goals.

**Embrace Balance:** Strive for balance in all aspects of your life, nurturing your body, mind, and soul with intention and care. Remember that health is not just about what you eat, but how you live each day with purpose and passion. cherish Life: Above all, cherish the gift of life and the beautiful moments that make it worth living. Find joy in the small pleasures, cherish the connections you share with loved ones, and savor each day as a wonderful opportunity to thrive.

As we bid adieu to your intermittent fasting journey, take a minute to express thanks for the experiences shared, the lessons learned, and the transformations achieved. May your road forward be filled with health, happiness, and many blessings, as you continue to embark on the adventure of a lifetime, One filled with vitality, purpose, and the infinite potential of the human spirit.

## Tips for Sustaining Your Progress: Maintaining Your Momentum

Congratulations on reaching the completion of your intermittent fasting journey! As you transition into the next chapter of your health and wellness adventure, it's crucial to incorporate tactics that will help you sustain the gains you've achieved and continue thriving in the long term. Here are some recommendations to help you keep your momentum and expand upon the great changes you've achieved:

**Establish Healthy Habits**: Intermittent fasting has provided you with a good basis for building healthy habits, such as mindful eating, regular physical activity, and stress management skills. Continue prioritizing these habits in your daily life, implementing them into your routine with consistency and determination.

**Make Realistic Goals:** As you move forward, make realistic and achievable goals that correspond with your values, priorities, and lifestyle. Break larger ambitions into smaller, attainable steps, and celebrate each milestone along the way. By setting specific targets and tracking your progress, you'll keep inspired and focused on your path.

**Stay Consistent:** Consistency is crucial to continuing your development over time. Stick to your established routines and habits, especially when faced with trials or disappointments. Remember that progress may not always be linear, but by keeping persistent and devoted to your goals, you'll continue moving forward on your journey to optimal health and wellness.

**Practice Mindful Eating:** Mindful eating entails paying attention to your body's hunger and fullness cues, as well as your food choices and eating patterns. Practice mindful eating strategies such as slowing down during meals, savoring each bite, and listening to your body's signals of hunger and satiety. By establishing a thoughtful approach to eating, you'll enrich your connection with food and support your long-term health goals.

**Prioritize Self-Care:** Self-care is vital for sustaining your physical, mental, and emotional well-being. Make time for things that nourish your body, mind, and spirit, whether it's practicing yoga, spending time outdoors, or indulging in a beloved pastime. Remember that self-care is not selfish, It's a necessary component of a balanced and satisfying existence.

**Seek Support:** Surround yourself with a supportive network of friends, family, or like-minded persons who can offer encouragement, guidance, and accountability on your journey. Share your objectives and challenges with others, and enjoy your triumphs together. By developing a sense of community and connection, you'll feel supported and empowered to sustain your success over the long term.

**Embrace Flexibility:** While consistency is vital, it's equally essential to embrace flexibility and adaptability in your approach to health and wellness. Life is full of unexpected twists and turns, and it's normal to change your plans and habits as needed. Be open to attempting new techniques, exploring other pathways, and adapting to changing conditions along the road.

**Practice thankfulness:** Cultivate an attitude of thankfulness for the progress you've made and the gifts in your life. Take time each day to reflect on the positive parts of your trip, show thanks for your achievements, and enjoy the minor wins. By focusing on appreciation, you'll nurture a good mindset and boost your overall sense of well-being.

**Monitor Your Progress:** Stay proactive in monitoring your progress and reviewing your findings often. Keep track of key variables such as weight, energy levels, mood, and overall health indicators to assess your progress and find areas for improvement. By keeping educated and proactive, you'll be more ready to make informed judgments and alter your strategy as needed.

**Stay Educated:** Finally, continue to educate yourself on health, wellness, and the newest research in the field. Stay updated about new discoveries, trends, and best practices, and be open to learning from experts, peers, and reputable sources. By keeping educated and informed, you'll empower yourself to make informed decisions and take proactive efforts toward enhancing your health and well-being.

As you bid farewell to your intermittent fasting journey and begin on the next part of your health and wellness adventure, remember that preserving your progress is a lifelong journey packed with possibilities for growth, learning, and self-discovery. By applying these advice and tactics, you'll be well-equipped to retain your momentum, overcome hurdles, and continue thriving on your path to optimal health and wellness. So, embrace the adventure with confidence, stay devoted to your goals, and keep pushing forward with courage and determination!

## Looking Ahead to a Healthy and Vibrant Future: Embracing Optimism

As you reach the completion of your intermittent fasting adventure, it's time to cast your focus forward and visualize the bright and vivid future that awaits you. In this segment, we'll cover the benefits of adopting optimism, creating objectives, and maintaining a positive mindset as you continue your journey toward maximum health and wellness.

## Embracing Optimism:

**Focus on opportunities:** Instead of concentrating on past struggles or setbacks, shift your focus to the boundless opportunities that lay ahead. Approach each day with a sense of optimism and enthusiasm, knowing that every moment is an opportunity for growth, transformation, and rejuvenation. Believe in Yourself: Cultivate self-belief and confidence in your capacity to overcome challenges and achieve your goals. Trust in your abilities, talents, and resilience, knowing that you have the capacity to create the future you wish.

**Stay Open to Opportunities:** Keep an open mind and heart as you traverse your health and wellness path, keeping attentive to new ideas, experiences, and possibilities for improvement. Embrace the unknown with curiosity and excitement, understanding that each obstacle is an opportunity for learning and expansion.

**Practice thankfulness:** Cultivate an attitude of thankfulness for the benefits in your life, concentrating on the abundance and positivity that surrounds you. Take time each day to think about the things you're thankful for, no matter how big or small, and embrace the beauty of the current moment.

**Stay Mindful:** Practice mindfulness and presence in your daily life, remaining sensitive to the present moment and completely participating in each experience as it unfolds.

Cultivate awareness of your thoughts, feelings, and sensations, and choose to respond with compassion and kindness. Surround Yourself with Positivity: Surround yourself with positive influences, including helpful friends, inspiring role models, and uplifting places. Seek out sources of inspiration and motivation that fire your spirit energize your soul, and separate yourself from negativity and pessimism.

As you bid farewell to your intermittent fasting journey and embark on the next chapter of your health and wellness adventure, remember to embrace the trip with positivity, establish goals for success, and create a positive mindset that propels you ahead. By imagining a healthy and bright future, setting clear intentions, and staying devoted to your goals, you'll create the life of your dreams and enjoy the endless possibilities that await you. So, look ahead with optimism, embrace the trip with an open heart, and let your dazzling soul illuminate the road to a future full of health, pleasure, and energy!

www.ingramcontent.com/pod-product-compliance
Lightning Source LLC
Chambersburg PA
CBHW050804250726
48653CB00006B/2070